Viral Infectious Diseases Annual Volume 2025

Edited by Shailendra K. Saxena

Published in London, United Kingdom

Viral Infectious Diseases Annual Volume 2025
http://dx.doi.org/10.5772/intechopen.1011164
Edited by Shailendra K. Saxena

Contributors
Abubakar Adamu, Ahmet Doğan, Arpita S. Harnam, Bariş Otlu, Bukhari ISah Shuaib, Evans Tumawu, Festus Agbatey, Godwin Amponsah Asiamah, Guodong Liang, Hari Kishan, Harry-César Ntumba Kayembe, Helena Quayson, Jean-Marie Ntumba Kayembe, Jinlin Wang, Jitesh Yadav, Karen Pomeyie, Lu Ga, Olamide Smart Aiyedogbon, Omosigho Omoruyi Pius, Prince Amoah Barnie, Ruijuan Li, Shailendra K. Saxena, Solomon Jonathan Hussaini, Taoran Wang, Timothy Adejoh Attah, Usman Aliyu Dutsinma, William Gyamesi, Xin Gao, Yan Huang, Yan Zhao, Yasemin Ersoy Çinar, Yihui Jin, Yuheng Ma, Yunfeng Xiao, Yuting Zhao, Çiğdem Kuzucu

First published in London, United Kingdom, 2026 by IntechOpen
IntechOpen is the global imprint of INTECHOPEN LIMITED, registered in England and Wales, registration number: 11086078, 167-169 Great Portland Street, London, W1W 5PF, United Kingdom

For EU product safety concerns: IN TECH d.o.o., Prolaz Marije Krucifikse Kozulić 3, 51000 Rijeka, Croatia, info@intechopen.com or visit our website at intechopen.com.

British Library Cataloguing-in-Publication Data
A catalogue record for this book is available from the British Library

Viral Infectious Diseases Annual Volume 2025
Edited by Shailendra K. Saxena
p. cm.

This title is part of the Infectious Diseases Book Series, Volume 45
Series Editor: Alfonso J. Rodriguez-Morales

Print ISBN 978-1-83635-989-0
Online ISBN 978-1-83635-988-3
eBook (PDF) ISBN 978-1-83635-990-6
ISSN 2631-6188

If disposing of this product, please recycle the paper responsibly.

IntechOpen Book Series

Infectious Diseases

Volume 45

Aims and Scope of the Series

This series will provide a comprehensive overview of recent research trends in various Infectious Diseases (as per the most recent Baltimore classification). Topics will include general overviews of infections, immunopathology, diagnosis, treatment, epidemiology, etiology, and current clinical recommendations for managing infectious diseases. Ongoing issues, recent advances, and future diagnostic approaches and therapeutic strategies will also be discussed. This book series will focus on various aspects and properties of infectious diseases whose deep understanding is essential for safeguarding the human race from losing resources and economies due to pathogens.

Meet the Series Editor

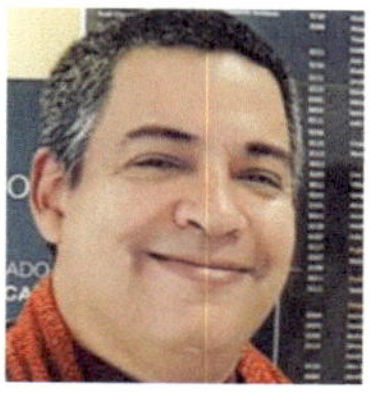

Dr. Alfonso J. Rodriguez-Morales received his MD from Universidad Central de Venezuela in Caracas and his MSc in Protozoology/Parasitology from Universidad de Los Andes in Trujillo, Venezuela. He received his Diploma in Tropical Medicine & Hygiene (DT-M&H) from Universidad Peruana Cayetano Heredia, Lima, Peru, and the University of Alabama at Birmingham, Alabama, USA. He also holds a DipEd. Dr. Rodriguez-Morales is a fellow of the Royal Society for Tropical Medicine & Hygiene (FRSTMH), London, United Kingdom; of the Faculty of Travel Medicine (FFTM) of the Royal College of Physicians and Surgeons of Glasgow (RCPSG), Glasgow, Scotland, United Kingdom; of the American College of Epidemiology (FACE), USA; and the International Society for Antimicrobial Chemotherapy (FISAC). He has a HonDSc from Universidad Privada Franz Tamayo (UniFranz), Cochabamba, Bolivia. He is the President of the Latin American Society for Travel Medicine (SLAMVI) (2023-2025) and the Past President of the Colombian Infectious Diseases Association (2021–2023). He is a member of the Council (2020-2026) of the International Society for Infectious Diseases (ISID). He is a senior researcher at Colciencias (2015–2027) and a professor at the Fundación Universitaria Autónoma de las Américas in Pereira, Risaralda, Colombia, as well as at the Universidad Científica del Sur (UCSUR) in Lima, Peru. He is a visiting professor at multiple national and international universities.

Meet the Volume Editor

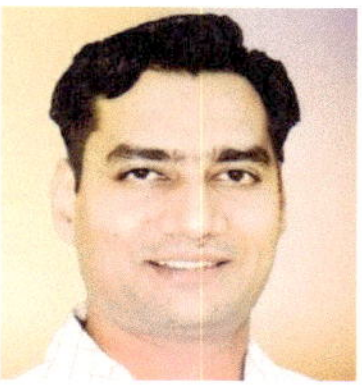

Professor Dr. Shailendra K. Saxena is a globally recognized biomedical scientist, serving as Vice Dean and distinguished Professor & Head at King George's Medical University (KGMU), Lucknow, India. Over several decades, he has emerged as a leading authority in biomedical sciences, molecular biology, and translational medicine, making landmark contributions to understanding viral infections and their neurological consequences. His research bridges fundamental science and practical healthcare, addressing complex medical challenges and advancing the United Nations Sustainable Development Goals by promoting health equity and global scientific awareness. His research interests include understanding the molecular mechanisms of host defense during human viral infections and developing new predictive, preventive, and therapeutic strategies for these infections using Japanese encephalitis virus (JEV), HIV, and emerging viruses as models, using stem cell and cell culture technologies. He gained international prominence during the COVID-19 pandemic by authoring the first comprehensive book on the disease and leading the world's first detailed analysis of the Omicron variant, informing WHO policies and global vaccination strategies. His research work has been published in various high-impact-factor journals. He has received many awards and honors in India and abroad, including the Young Scientist Awards, the BBSRC India Partnering Award, and the Dr. JC Bose National Award from the Department of Biotechnology, Ministry of Science and Technology, Govt. of India. Dr. Saxena is a fellow of various prestigious international societies/academies, including the Royal College of Pathologists, United Kingdom; the Royal Society of Medicine, London; the Royal Society of Biology, United Kingdom; the Royal Society of Chemistry, London; and the Academy of Translational Medicine Professionals, Austria. Named a Global Leader in Science by The Scientist, an international opinion leader on Japanese encephalitis vaccination, a Clarivate Highly Cited Researcher, a ScholarGPS™ Highly Ranked Scholar (Top 0. 05% Lifetime), and among Stanford University's "World's Top 2% Scientists," he exemplifies integrating cutting-edge science with societal impact, advancing global health, and fostering world peace through innovation, collaboration, and practical healthcare solutions.

Contents

Preface

The relationship between humans and viruses is as ancient as civilization itself. Early depictions in Egyptian hieroglyphs from around 3700 BC, illustrating paralytic deformities and variolous lesions, attest to humanity's longstanding encounters with poliomyelitis and smallpox. However, despite millennia of observation, viruses remained scientifically enigmatic until the late 19th century, when advances in filtration and microscopy confirmed their existence and ushered in the modern discipline of virology. By the mid-20th century, more than 2,000 viral species had been identified, marking an exceptional period of scientific progress. Despite these advances, viral pathogens continue to evolve with remarkable speed. Modern outbreaks, shaped by zoonotic spillover, increased human mobility, and ecological disruption, underscore the persistent and unpredictable nature of viral diseases. Epidemics today demonstrate considerable heterogeneity in severity, duration, recurrence, and clinical burden, influenced by viral mutation dynamics, host immune responses, environmental pressures, and disparities in health systems. Vulnerable populations, including infants, young children, immunocompromised individuals, and adults in their most productive years, remain disproportionately affected.

Scientific progress in molecular biology, sequencing technologies, structural virology, and computational modelling has deepened our understanding of viral evolution and host–pathogen interactions. However, the rapid adaptability of viruses, particularly RNA viruses with high mutation rates, continues to challenge existing therapeutic and preventive strategies. Drug resistance, immune escape mechanisms, and the persistence of latent reservoirs remain major concerns for global health. The repeated emergence of highly pathogenic viruses, ranging from novel coronaviruses and expanding arboviruses to drug-resistant HIV, HBV, and HCV variants, highlights the need for sustained, coordinated global action. A multidisciplinary approach involving basic scientists, clinicians, epidemiologists, regulatory authorities, public health experts, and the broader community is essential to address these evolving threats. Strengthening research capacity through enhanced laboratory infrastructure, biosafety systems, and advanced academic training remains critical to support high-quality virological research and preparedness.

Although diagnostic technologies have advanced significantly, the availability of targeted antiviral therapies and vaccines for many emerging viruses remains limited. The rise of drug-resistant strains further complicates clinical management. Continued innovation in antiviral discovery, immunotherapy, and vaccine development, along with the growing promise of precision medicine informed by host and viral genomics, is vital to improving global outcomes. The chapters in this volume reflect the breadth and complexity of contemporary research on viral infectious diseases. They offer critical insights into HIV neuropathogenesis, drug resistance evolution under HAART pressure, and global strategies to enhance viral suppression among people living with HIV. Additional contributions address advances in peptide-based fusion inhibitors and the epidemiology and management of atypical and viral pneumonias, including in resource-limited settings. Together, these works illuminate key scientific, clinical, and public health dimensions of viral disease management.

This volume forms an integral part of the *Infectious Diseases Book Series*, which seeks to provide a rigorous, forward-looking synthesis of emerging trends, research innovations, and strategic priorities in virology. The collective efforts of contributing authors, expert reviewers, mentors, and supporting colleagues have greatly enriched this work. Their dedication is deeply appreciated, and their contributions advance our shared mission of strengthening global responses to viral infectious diseases.

Shailendra K. Saxena
Centre for Advanced Research,
Faculty of Medicine,
King George's Medical University,
Lucknow, India

Dedicated to my parents & family who believed in academics as the way forward for an intelligent mind and to the teachers who introduced me the subject and nurtured my interest in it.

Section 1

Global Challenges and Therapeutic Advances – HIV and NeuroAIDS

Chapter 1

Therapeutic Advances and Challenges in NeuroAIDS Management in the cART Era toward Global Strategies

Jitesh Yadav, Arpita S. Harnam, Hari Kishan and Shailendra K. Saxena

Abstract

Despite the transformative impact of combination antiretroviral therapy (cART) in improving survival and systemic viral suppression, human immunodeficiency virus (HIV) continues to pose major global health challenges, particularly through its persistent effects on the central nervous system (CNS). The neurological complications associated with HIV, collectively termed neuroAIDS, remain a significant clinical concern due to the CNS's role as a reservoir for latent infection. This sanctuary status is facilitated by the restrictive nature of the blood-brain barrier and the long-lived persistence of infected microglia, macrophages, astrocytes, and resting CD4+ T cells. Mechanisms of viral entry into the CNS—such as the "Trojan Horse" hypothesis and direct transcytosis—enable early seeding of the brain, complicating long-term viral eradication efforts. While antiretroviral therapy (ART) regimens with higher CNS penetration effectiveness (CPE) scores are generally more successful in suppressing cerebrospinal fluid (CSF) viral loads, neurotoxicity associated with some high-CPE agents underscores the delicate balance between efficacy and safety. Therapeutic challenges also include incomplete CNS drug penetration, the evolution of compartmentalized drug-resistant viral variants, and adverse interactions with treatments for comorbid conditions, all of which limit full neurocognitive recovery. This chapter reviews the recent therapeutic advances aimed at overcoming these barriers, including intensified ART regimens, CCR5 antagonists, nanoparticle-based CNS drug delivery, gene-editing strategies, neuroprotective interventions, and immunomodulatory therapies. By examining these emerging approaches through a global health lens, we explore their potential to inform more effective, accessible, and sustainable strategies for the management of neuroAIDS—ultimately progressing toward the goal of long-term remission and a functional cure.

Keywords: NeuroAIDS, CNS penetration-effectiveness (CPE), antiretroviral therapy (ART), HIV-associated neurocognitive disorders (HAND), neuroprotection in HIV

1. Introduction

Human immunodeficiency virus (HIV) is a retrovirus that attacks the immune system, CD4+ T cells, and causes progressive immunodeficiency. Acquired immunodeficiency syndrome (AIDS) is a very late stage of the HIV infection, which is extremely immunosuppressed and vulnerable to opportunistic diseases and cancer. By 2024, there will be about 39 million individuals residing with HIV across the world, and it is estimated that 630,000 deaths related to AIDs will occur within the same year, notwithstanding the excellent advancements in prevention, testing, and treatment interventions. The virus is spread by the means of certain body fluids such as blood, semen, vaginal secretions, and breast milk and may also be transferred by mother to child during pregnancy, childbirth, or breastfeeding. Hugging, kissing, or sharing food do not aid transmission since it is casual. Combination antiretroviral therapy (cART) is the most significant way of managing HIV infection and thereby slowing down the progression of the disease by inhibiting the synthesis of the virus and also restoring the immune system. The current definition of advanced HIV disease (AHD) as provided by the World Health Organization (WHO) is a CD4+ cell count below 200 cells/mm^3 or the occurrence of WHO clinical stage 3 or 4 ailments in adults and adolescents. Moreover, children less than 5 years old who have HIV are all considered to have an advanced HIV disease since they are more susceptible [1]. NeuroAIDS is a term used to describe the range of neurological conditions linked to HIV infection. These complications comprise cognitive, motor, and behavioral dysfunctions, which occur as the virus affects the central and peripheral nervous systems [2]. It includes conditions such as HIV-associated neurocognitive disorders (HAND) and HIV-associated dementia (HAD), manifested through cognitive and motor disabilities caused by the effects of HIV on the central nervous system [3]. Other symptoms are peripheral neuropathies, opportunistic infections (tuberculous and cryptococcal meningitis), and AIDS dementia complex [4]. HIV/AIDS management is based on antiretroviral therapy (ART), a combination of medications meant to interfere with various HIV life cycle stages. Its main objective is to inhibit viral replication, rebuild and maintain immune activity, and prevent morbidity and death related to HIV. The cART, previously referred to as highly active antiretroviral therapy (HAART), has played an incredible role in reducing the prevalence of AIDS-defining conditions, including neurological complications like AIDS dementia complex (ADC) and HIV-associated neurocognitive disorders (HAND). ART is not only associated with decreased plasma viral load but also with reduced HIV replication in the central nervous system (CNS), resulting in improved neurological function and a significant decrease in opportunistic infections of the CNS [5–7].

2. Pathophysiology of neuroAIDS

2.1 Mechanisms of HIV entry into the CNS

HIV is a neurotropic virus and can penetrate the brain in 1–2 weeks following its systemic infection. Despite the availability of HAART, HIV disease still continues to prevail in the CNS, and CNS-related neurological issues are still present [8]. HIV can evade the intense blood-brain barrier (BBB) and enter the brain (**Figure 1**). Major pathways proposed for HIV entry into the brain (**Table 1**).

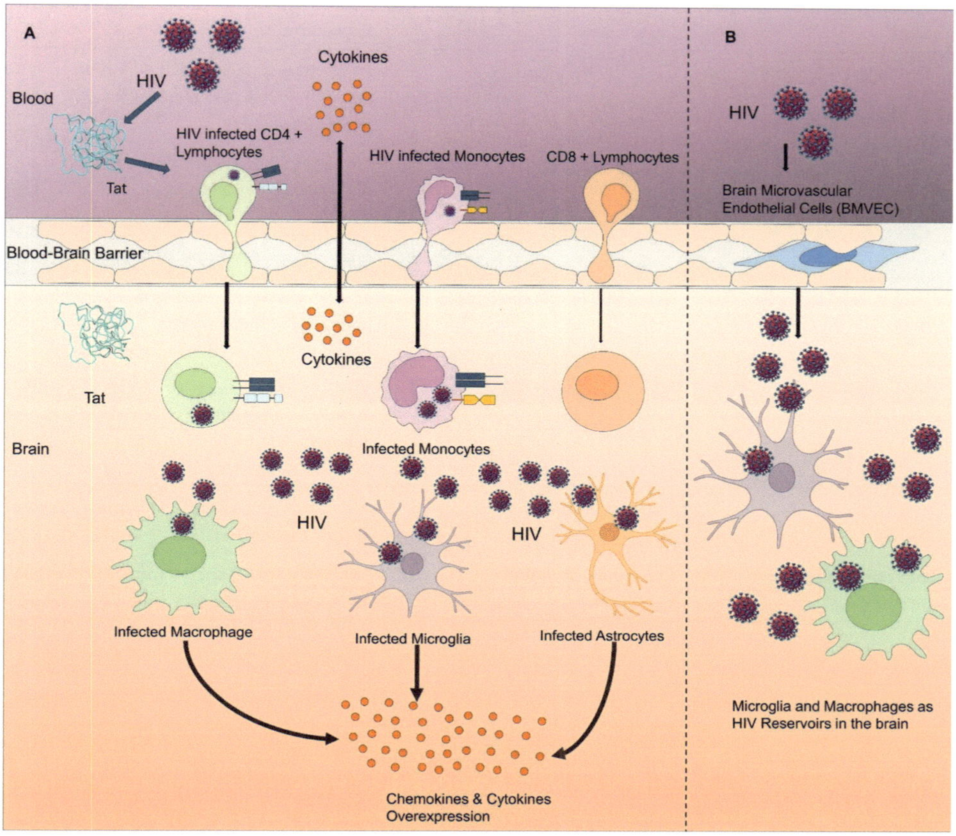

Figure 1.
Mechanisms of HIV entry into the CNS and establishment of viral reservoirs in the brain. (A) The mechanisms by which HIV crosses the blood-brain barrier (BBB). In the periphery, HIV infects CD4+ T lymphocytes and monocytes, which releases viral proteins such as Tat and inflammatory cytokines. These HIV-infected monocytes and lymphocytes migrate across the BBB, aided by BBB disruption and cytokine signaling, and differentiate into infected macrophages within the brain parenchyma. (B) Establishes persistent viral reservoirs in the central nervous system (CNS). Another way HIV crosses the BBB is via brain microvascular endothelial cells (BMVEC) through transcytosis. Once within the CNS, HIV infects resident microglia, macrophages, and astrocytes, which acts as long-lived viral reservoirs. These infected glial cells contribute to chronic neuroinflammation through sustained production of chemokines and cytokines, exacerbating neuronal dysfunction and contributing to the development of HIV-associated neurocognitive disorders (HAND).

2.1.1 Trojan Horse hypothesis

This hypothesis proposes that the brain becomes infected as HIV-infected immune cells, particularly monocytes and lymphocytes, migrate across the BBB [9]. HIV-infected monocytes and T-lymphocytes have been hypothesized to be important in the transfer of HIV into the CNS. Various adhesion molecules, tight junction proteins, and chemokine receptors are expressed to a higher degree in the HIV infected monocytes (CD14+ and CD16+), facilitating their transmigration into the CNS [10].

2.1.2 Cell-free virus entry into CNS

The HIV components in the blood can penetrate the brain through the brain microvascular endothelial cells (BMVEC), which form the BBB, can internalize HIV

Step	Performers	Procedure
Peripheral infection	$CD4^+$ T cells, monocytes	HIV infects circulating $CD4^+$ T-lymphocytes and monocytes, and releases Tat and cytokines
BBB crossing	Infected monocytes ("Trojan Horse")	Monocytes transmigrate into the CNS *via* disrupted tight junctions (occludin/ZO-1)
Cell-free transcytosis	HIV virions, BMVEC	Direct uptake and transcytosis through brain microvascular endothelial cells
Differentiation in the brain	Monocyte → macrophage	Transmigrated monocytes differentiate into perivascular macrophages, and harbor latent virus
Infection of resident glia	Microglia, astrocytes	Virus spreads to microglia and astrocytes; astrocyte infection *via* endocytosis or cell-cell contact
Reservoir establishment	Microglia, macrophages, astrocytes, and memory $CD4^+$ T cells	Long-lived cells maintain a latent provirus and can reactivate under inflammatory/ immune stimuli
Neuroinflammatory amplification	Cytokines, chemokines, and viral proteins	Infected glia releases inflammatory mediators and exosomes → neuronal injury → HAND

Table 1.
Mechanisms of HIV entry into the CNS and reservoir establishment.

particles into intracellular vacuoles, and transport them across the BBB *via* transcytosis. Although BMVECs typically lack CD4 receptors, HIV entry occurs through alternative pathways such as adsorptive endocytosis mediated by gp120. However, the majority (over 99%) of the internalized virus is subsequently degraded in lysosomes, with less than 1% successfully traversing the endothelial layer to reach the brain parenchyma [11]. BMVECs usually do not express CD4 receptors, and the entry of HIV into these cells is not blocked by chemokines or CD4-targeting inhibitors. Other cell surface molecules, such as the C-type lectins DC-SIGN and L-SIGN, and cell-surface proteoglycans, are more likely to mediate HIV attachment and entry [12]. Despite this, the majority of the virus internalized in the BMVECs is degraded in lysosomes, and it is believed that fewer than 1 percent of the virus that gets through successfully crosses the BMVEC layer [13].

2.2 HIV reservoirs and viral persistence in the brain

Some of the HIV reservoirs in the body include the brain and the gut, where the virus may remain despite ART. This survival makes it difficult to cure HIV because the infection returns rapidly when treatment is not continually followed or discontinued [8]. A virus might remain in the gut due to certain genetic variations among the various sections of the gut [14]. Similarly, HIV can also become compartmentalized in the brain, and the virus can evolve in the same way, which allows the virus to escape the clearance mechanism of the body. This gives rise to a different form of a virus that can only multiply in the case of a weak immune system [15]. In CNS, HIV infects both microglia and monocyte-derived macrophages that serve as key cellular reservoirs, producing inflammatory mediators like IL-18, IL-1β, and caspase-1 *via* NLRP3 inflammasome activation, contributing to neuroinflammation and neuronal damage [16]. HIV susceptible macrophages and microglia migrate to the site of infection and release inflammatory superoxide due to the HIV negative regulatory factor (Nef) protein [17].

Monocytes that enter the CNS to differentiate into macrophages undergo β-catenin downregulation, making them more susceptible to HIV infection [18]. HIV-infected macrophages resist apoptosis and immune clearance, maintaining latent infection under ART, with factors like leukotriene C4 facilitating infected CD4+ T cell trafficking into the brain and viral spread to resident macrophages and microglia [19, 20]. Astrocytes, the most abundant glial cells in the brain, despite a low HIV integration rate (0.1–1%), constitute a significant reservoir due to their abundance, confirmed by techniques such as *in situ* hybridization and RNA/DNA scope [21]. Infected astrocytes disrupt the BBB, impair gap junctions, and drive neuroinflammation *via* altered β-catenin signaling, while latency-reversing agents (LRAs) can reactivate HIV within them [22, 23]. Astrocytes can also transfer HIV to CD4+ T cells, potentially reseeding peripheral infection during treatment interruptions. Though lacking classic HIV entry receptors, astrocytes acquire HIV through pH-dependent endocytosis or direct contact with infected T cells [24, 25]. HIV is primarily maintained in a small fraction (<0.05%) of resting CD4+ T cells, particularly long-lived memory CD4+ T cells, which harbors an integrated but transcriptionally silent HIV-1 provirus. Despite their low frequency, these cells represent a major obstacle to viral eradication. Naive CD4+ T cells are generally CCR5-negative, while memory CD4+ T cell subsets can express variable levels of both CCR5 and CXCR4, with CCR5 expression particularly associated with the activated and effector memory subsets. Memory CD4+ T cells are especially suited to maintain latency due to their longevity and quiescent state, which supports minimal viral transcription and evades immune detection. These cells can produce low levels of virus, potentially reseeding infection, and can reactivate under immune stimulation [26].

3. Antiretroviral therapy (ART) for neuroAIDS

The most conventional treatment of HIV infection is through ART. It implies a combination of drugs that act on various stages of the HIV life cycle with the aim of inhibiting viral replication, lowering viral load, and restoring immune function. Standard ART regimens for neuroAIDS have historically included two nucleoside analogues (NAs), such as zidovudine or stavudine, which were among the first agents shown to penetrate the CSF and exert a beneficial effect on HIV-associated brain disease. However, due to the significant long-term toxicities, including mitochondrial toxicity and bone marrow suppression, these agents have largely been phased out of modern treatment protocols. Contemporary guidelines now favor better-tolerated NRTIs such as tenofovir and emtricitabine or lamivudine. Protease inhibitors (PIs) have been variably used for CNS protection, though their value remains under evaluation. Non-nucleoside reverse transcriptase inhibitors (NNRTIs), particularly nevirapine and efavirenz, were historically regarded as CNS-active agents. While combinations of two NAs and one NNRTI were once widely recommended, modern first-line regimens now prioritize integrase strand transfer inhibitors (INSTIs) due to their superior efficacy, tolerability, and favorable CNS penetration profiles. Nevertheless, historical regimens and their CNS penetration data remain relevant in understanding neuroAIDS management evolution and guiding care in resource-limited settings where older drugs may still be in use [27].

The application of ART has revolutionized the process of managing HIV and its related neurological disorders, collectively referred to as neuroAIDS. With the advent of HAART, the CNS has emerged as a key sanctuary site of HIV-1, thus rendering CNS-active ART regimens as crucial determinants of prophylaxis and treatment of HAND and AIDS dementia complex (ADC) [28].

A combination of two NAs and one NNRTI is usually suggested, particularly among patients with high plasma viral loads and some abnormalities of the neurologic system. But it is accompanied by a subpopulation of non-responders who have to be offered other or supplementary treatments [28].

The success of using ART in the treatment of neuroAIDS is closely correlated with the capacity of antiretroviral drugs to cross the CNS barrier. This will be quantified through CNS penetration effectiveness (CPE) score, which is used to rank ART drugs in terms of chemical properties, CSF concentrations, and clinical efficacy in the CNS. The CNS penetration values of each ART drug come out as a CPE score of between 1 (below average) and 4 (much above average). Higher cumulative CPE score drugs (zidovudine, nevirapine, and ritonavir-boosted indinavir) are linked to interventions that result in better suppression of HIV in the CSF, while poor CNS penetration permits further replication of HIV in the CNS, which results in increased CSF HIV viral loads and possibly poorer neurocognitive outcomes [29, 30].

Although higher CPE regimens are usually associated with better CSF virus suppression, there are inconsistent results on their effects on neuropsychological performance. Other high-CNS penetrating regimens have been linked to worse neuropsychological results, which might exist due to neurotoxicity of some agents. The correlation between CSF drug concentrations and those of the actual brain tissue is not well understood, and there are mechanisms through which drugs can be restricted from gaining access to the brain, for example, protein pump (e.g., P-glycoprotein) [29]. Adjunctive therapies are also under investigation to target neuroinflammation and neuroprotection, although none have so far consistently shown clinical benefit in large studies.

4. Challenges in ART for neuroAIDS

Inadequate penetration of drugs into the CNS remains a major therapeutic challenge in managing neuroAIDS, as the BBB restricts many agents from achieving effective concentrations in CSF. Certain classes of efflux transporters, such as those of P-glycoprotein, MRP, and BCRP, actively pump drugs such as ritonavir and saquinavir out of the brain, and physicochemical characteristics such as increased molecular size and reduced lipophilicity further impede passive diffusion. For instance, tenofovir disoproxil fumarate achieves CSF concentrations of less than 7 ng/mL, a fraction of its plasma concentration, which may be insufficient for optimal viral suppression in the CNS. Although regimens with greater CPE scores can enhance suppression of CSF viral loads, clinical benefits remain inconsistent, and neurotoxicity risks from certain high-CPE agents persist, for example, efavirenz [31, 32]. This limited entry enables HIV reservoirs to exist in microglia and perivascular macrophages, supporting low-level viral replication and clonal expansion. Compounding this issue, subtherapeutic levels of ART in the CNS promote the independent evolution of HIV-1, predisposing the selection of resistance mutations that subsequently can expand systemically. Concordant resistance mutations have been reported in CSF and plasma to protease inhibitors (PIs), nucleoside reverse transcriptase inhibitors (NRTIs), and non-nucleoside reverse transcriptase inhibitors (NNRTIs), with ART itself an increasing risk factor for CSF resistance (OR = 4.25) because of partial suppression [33]. Also, long-term ART treatment is the cause of CNS complications through mitochondrial disease since NRTIs such as zidovudine block mitochondrial DNA polymerase-γ, which causes oxidative stress and neuronal damage, whereas protease inhibitors, like darunavir, disintegrate the BBB, triggering microglia, increasing the levels of neurofilament light chains in CSF. Efavirenz is a notable example, associated with neuropsychiatric adverse effects including depression, hallucinations, and vivid dreams in up to 40% of patients, particularly during the early phases of treatment or in antiretroviral-naïve individuals. These effects are thought to be mediated through NMDA receptor modulation and serotonergic pathways, and while often transient, can lead to poor adherence or necessitate regimen changes in the affected individuals. Drug-drug interactions and co-infections further complicate the management of neuroAIDS; ritonavir-enhanced regimens have the effect of inhibiting CYP3A4, thereby increasing the neurotoxic levels of drugs such as sertraline and anticonvulsants. Other risks include co-infections like tuberculosis, whereby rifampicin reduces the nevirapine concentrations by 37%, which leads to the increased risk of virologic failure in the CNS, and hepatitis C co-infection that complicates ART because of the risk of hepatotoxicity and neuroinflammation caused by HCV that aggravates HIV-associated neurocognitive disorders (HAND). The continued inflammation in the CNS with the development of ART, evidenced in elevated CSF myoinositol/creatinine ratios, also makes the effective treatment of neuroAIDS complicated due to these co-morbidities [31, 32]. ART challenges and emerging neuroAIDS strategies are shown in **Table 2**.

5. Recent advances and emerging strategies

Although the introduction of cART in managing HIV disease has transformed the disease by improving life expectancy, there are still many challenges in managing HIV-related neurological comorbidities (neuroAIDS). These challenges involve the existence of the CNS as the viral reservoir, the BBB obstacle to successful pharmaceutical entry, and chronic neuroinflammation and neurotoxicity despite the viral suppression [34]. In response to these persistent issues, recent advances and emerging strategies in ART for neuroAIDS focus on improving cART efficacy within the CNS, developing novel drug delivery methods, repurposing existing drugs to target downstream neuropathogenesis, and exploring the non-pharmacological interventions.

Class	Barrier	Emerging strategy
CNS drug penetration	Efflux transporters (P-gp, MRP, BCRP); low lipophilicity	Nanoparticle-based ART; cell-mediated nanoART
	CPE score limitations	Optimized formulations; ligand-targeted BBB transport
Latent reservoirs	Persistent virus in glial cells	"Shock-and-kill" (LRAs); "Block-and-lock" approaches
Neurotoxicity	High-CPE agent side effects (efavirenz, DTG)	Neuroprotective adjuvants, dose adjustments, and drug repurposing
Drug resistance	Compartmentalized resistance in CSF vs. plasma	Next-gen INSTIs; combination intensification; CCR5/CCR2 blockade
Neuroinflammation	Chronic glial activation; cytokine storms	CCR5/CCR2 antagonists; JAK inhibitors; immunomodulators
Innovative therapies	Safety and delivery challenges (gene editing, immunotherapy)	CRISPR/Cas9; therapeutic vaccines; broadly neutralizing Abs

Table 2.
ART challenges and emerging neuroAIDS strategies.

5.1 Enhancing CNS penetrance

In recent ART advances, drug penetration into the CNS has been approached by improving the passage of drugs through the BBB to achieve better drug access to HIV reservoirs in the CNS. The concept of CPE scores has been developed to rank antiretroviral drugs based on their ability to penetrate the BBB. While the clinical significance of CPE in terms of reducing HAND symptoms is not entirely clear, and some studies show paradoxical associations, some evidence suggests that higher CPE may correlate with better CNS HIV suppression and potential benefits for HIV-associated neurocognitive impairment (HIV-NCI) [34]. Newer integrase strand transfer inhibitors (INSTIs), including elvitegravir, have shown better CNS penetration, particularly when given in an enhanced delivery formulation [35, 36]. Second-generation INSTIs have become preferred in most first-line regimens, and a dose adjustment is being contemplated in the case of CNS resistance. However, the optimization of CNS penetration should be balanced with the risk of neurotoxicity, with a subset of high-penetrance agents (e.g., dolutegravir, efavirenz) leading to the neuropsychiatric adverse effects [35].

5.2 Chemokine receptor blockade

ART intensification with the use of the CCR5 chemokine receptor antagonist maraviroc, an HIV-entry inhibitor, was studied as a method of minimizing the risk of HIV-NCI. Pilot studies demonstrated the promising effects, with cognitive outcomes in virally suppressed people with HAND, with or without an associated improvement in inflammatory biomarkers. There is enthusiasm for CCR5 blockade in general neuroinflammatory disorders. The dual CCR2 and CCR5 antagonist cenicriviroc inhibits not only HIV infection but also inflammation and monocyte migration. In a pilot trial in virally suppressed individuals with mild-to-moderate HIV-NCI, small positive changes in neurocognitive performance and a reduction in plasma measures of monocyte activation markers were observed. The potential neuroprotective effects of blocking both CCR5 and CCR2 are being considered for larger studies [34].

5.3 Nanoparticle-based drug delivery

Nanoparticle-based drug delivery systems target to enhance the distribution of ARV drugs in the brain and have the following advantages: enhanced bioavailability, extended circulation time, and targeting capabilities [36]. Poloxamer-PLGA and nanodiamonds are the nanoparticles (NPs) that have been designed to deliver ART drugs such as efavirenz and elvitegravir across the BBB and exhibit greater uptake and inhibition of viruses *in vitro*, in HIV-infected macrophages, and *in vivo* [35, 37, 38]. Liposome-based nanomedicines play a critical role in the delivery of hydrophobic antiviral HIV drugs (i.e., zidovudine, zalcitabine, didanosine) across the BBB, and the stability and circulation of these drugs can be enhanced by making alterations such as PEGylation [39]. Magnetic nanoparticles (MNPs) such as magnetite ($Fe3O4$) and maghemite (γ-$Fe2O3$) provided the targeted drug delivery with the capacity of external guidance and simultaneous monitoring *via* MRI [39]. nanoART may also be *ex vivo* loaded into cell-mediated delivery mononuclear phagocytes (MP) such as dendritic cells, monocytes, and macrophages that once re-introduced to the body can cross the BBB and deposit drugs locally at sites of infection and can sustain the therapeutic levels of drugs in the CNS over prolonged periods of time [37]. This has been done with nanosuspensions of ritonavir and efavirenz [39]. To increase the uptake by

HIV-infected cells and increase specificity of targeting, NP surfaces are being modified with ligands (e.g., mannose, tuftsin) [40].

5.4 Targeting downstream pathways and repurposing existing drugs

Drugs like baricitinib (JAK1/2 inhibitor) have shown the ability to cross the BBB and reduce HIV persistence in the CNS in preclinical and early clinical studies, with ongoing trials assessing their impact on neurocognitive outcomes [41]. The neuroprotective agents (minocycline, selegiline, and statins) have been evaluated in their neuroprotective or anti-inflammatory properties, but clinical trials have not shown definite cognitive effects of drugs in HAND [35, 42]. Probiotic supplementation has shown early evidence of decreasing CSF neopterin concentration and improving neurocognitive performance in small pilot studies [34].

5.5 Gene therapy and immunotherapeutic approaches

CRISPR/Cas9 gene-editing technology is being explored to disrupt HIV proviral DNA or modify host genes such as CCR5 to confer resistance to infection. Early clinical trials have demonstrated the feasibility of infusing gene-edited immune cells to reduce viral loads and enhance resistance in patients. However, concerns regarding off-target effects, immune responses, and safety in CNS applications remain significant hurdles for clinical translation [43, 44]. Metabolic Therapies Shock-and-kill tactics employ latency-reversing agents (LRAs) to re-activate dormant HIV in CNS reservoirs, as well as subsequent eradication by immune responses or suicide gene therapy. However, the reactivation in the CNS can lead to unacceptable neuron injury and inflammation, and this factor presents a considerable safety issue [35, 43]. Additional strategies, including therapeutic vaccines, cytokine therapies (e.g., IL-7, IL-15, IL-21), broadly neutralizing antibodies, and immune checkpoint modulation, are also under investigation for their potential to augment immune clearance of infected cells within the CNS. Antibody-based therapies and immune checkpoint modulation are also being studied to enhance the immune system targeting HIV-infected cells [44, 45].

6. Conclusions

Despite remarkable advances in cART transforming HIV from a fatal disease into a manageable chronic infection in regions with consistent access to ART, significant challenges remain in addressing the neurological complications collectively known as neuroAIDS. The CNS serves as a critical viral reservoir, sheltering HIV within long-lived cells such as microglia, macrophages, astrocytes, and resting memory CD4+ T cells, where the virus persists in a latent state, often inaccessible to standard ART regimens. While higher CNS-penetrating antiretrovirals offer improved CSF viral suppression, their clinical impact on neurocognitive outcomes remains inconsistent, with certain high-penetrance agents associated with neurotoxicity. Persistent neuroinflammation, the emergence of drug-resistant viral variants within the CNS, and complex drug-drug interactions further complicate long-term management. However, recent advances in CNS-targeted drug delivery systems, such as nanoparticle-based formulations and cell-mediated therapies, alongside novel strategies such as CCR5 and CCR2 antagonism, gene-editing technologies, and immunomodulatory approaches, offer promising avenues to overcome these barriers. Moving forward, future strategies must focus on improving CNS drug bioavailability, effectively targeting latent reservoirs, mitigating chronic neuroinflammation, and integrating multimodal therapies to reduce the burden of HAND. A multidisciplinary, globally coordinated effort will be essential to refine therapeutic strategies, translate emerging interventions into clinical practice, and ultimately improve the quality of life and neurological health outcomes for people living with HIV.

7. Future perspectives

The management of neuroAIDS remains a significant challenge despite the success of cART. Future strategies must prioritize the development of antiretroviral agents with enhanced CNS penetration and minimized neurotoxicity, along with innovative drug delivery systems such as nanoparticle-based formulations to effectively target latent viral reservoirs within the brain. Promising avenues include gene-editing technologies, CCR5/CCR2 receptor antagonists, immunotherapies, and neuroprotective agents aimed at suppressing viral persistence and mitigating chronic neuroinflammation. The integration of these emerging interventions into personalized, CNS-focused treatment regimens should be supported by well-designed multicentric clinical trials and translational research programs to validate their safety, efficacy, and long-term impact on neurocognitive outcomes, ultimately advancing the field toward a functional cure for HIV.

Acknowledgements

The authors are grateful to the Vice Chancellor, King George's Medical University (KGMU), Lucknow, for the encouragement and support for this work. The authors have no other relevant affiliations or financial involvement with any organization or entity with a financial interest in or financial conflict with the subject matter or materials discussed in the manuscript apart from those disclosed.

Funding

This research did not receive any specific grant from funding agencies in the public, commercial, or not-for-profit sectors.

Conflict of interest

None.

Acronyms and abbreviations

ADC	AIDS dementia complex
AHD	Advanced HIV disease
ART	Antiretroviral therapy
BMVEC	Brain microvascular endothelial cells
BBB	Blood-brain barrier

CART	Combination antiretroviral therapy
CPE	CNS Penetration Effectiveness
CNS	Central nervous system
CSF	Cerebrospinal fluid
cART	Combination Antiretroviral Therapy
FIs	Fusion Inhibitors
HAND	HIV-associated neurocognitive disorders
HAART	Highly active antiretroviral therapy
HAD	HIV-associated dementia
HIV-NCI	HIV-associated neurocognitive impairment
INSTIs	Integrase strand transfer inhibitors
LRAs	Latency-reversing agents
MP	Mononuclear phagocytes
MNPs	Magnetic nanoparticles
MRP	Multidrug Resistance-associated Protein
NAs	Nucleoside analogues
NLRP3	NOD-, LRR- and Pyrin Domain-Containing Protein 3
NNRTIs	Non-nucleoside reverse transcriptase inhibitors
NRTIs	Nucleoside/Nucleotide Reverse Transcriptase Inhibitors
NPs	Nanoparticles
PIs	Protease inhibitors
PLGA	Poly (lactic-co-glycolic acid)
WHO	World Health Organization

Author details

Jitesh Yadav†, Arpita S. Harnam, Hari Kishan and Shailendra K. Saxena†*
Centre for Advanced Research (CFAR), Faculty of Medicine, King George's Medical University (KGMU), Lucknow, India

*Address all correspondence to: shailen@kgmcindia.edu

† Contributed equally to the chapter.

References

[1] World Health Organization. 2024. Available from: https://www.who.int/news-room/fact-sheets/detail/hiv-aids [Accessed: 19 June 2025]

[2] Rahimian P, He JJ. HIV/neuroAIDS biomarkers. Progress in Neurobiology. 2017;**157**:117-132. DOI: 10.1016/j.pneurobio.2016.04.003

[3] Minagar A, Commins D, Alexander JS, Hoque R, Chiappelli F, Singer EJ, et al. NeuroAIDS: Characteristics and diagnosis of the neurological complications of AIDS. Molecular Diagnosis & Therapy. 2008;**12**(1):25-43. DOI: 10.1007/BF03256266

[4] Bhagwat K, Yegade W, Singh J, Meshram A, Goel J. Study of clinical spectrum of neurological manifestations in HIV/AIDS seen at tertiary referral hospital in India. Vidarbha Journal of Internal Medicine. 2023;**33**:82-89. DOI: 10.25259/VJIM_5_2024

[5] Price RW, Spudich S. Antiretroviral therapy and central nervous system HIV type 1 infection. The Journal of Infectious Diseases. 2008;**197**:S294-S306. DOI: 10.1086/533419

[6] Ellis R, Letendre SL. Update and new directions in therapeutics for neurological complications of HIV infections. Neurotherapeutics. 2016;**13**(3):471-476. DOI: 10.1007/s13311-016-0454-2

[7] Saxena SK, Sharma D, Kumar S, Puri B. Understanding HIV-associated neurocognitive and neurodegenerative disorders (neuroAIDS): Enroute to achieve the 95-95-95 target and sustainable development goal for HIV/AIDS response. Virus. 2023;**34**(2):165-171. DOI: 10.1007/s13337-023-00830-1

[8] Ash MK, Al-Harthi L, Schneider JR. HIV in the brain: Identifying viral reservoirs and addressing the challenges of an HIV cure. Vaccines (Basel). 2021;**9**(8):867. DOI: 10.3390/vaccines9080867

[9] Marchetti L, Engelhardt B. Immune cell trafficking across the blood-brain barrier in the absence and presence of neuroinflammation. Vascular Biology. 2020;**2**(1):H1-H18. DOI: 10.1530/VB-19-0033

[10] Williams DW, Calderon TM, Lopez L, Carvallo-Torres L, Gaskill PJ, Eugenin EA, et al. Mechanisms of HIV entry into the CNS: Increased sensitivity of HIV infected CD14+CD16+ monocytes to CCL2 and key roles of CCR2, JAM-A, and ALCAM in diapedesis. PLoS One. 2013;**8**(7):e69270. DOI: 10.1371/journal.pone.0069270

[11] Banks WA, Kastin AJ, Brennan JM, Vallance KL. Adsorptive endocytosis of HIV-1gp120 by blood-brain barrier is enhanced by lipopolysaccharide. Experimental Neurology. 1999;**156**(1):165-171. DOI: 10.1006/exnr.1998.7011

[12] Argyris EG, Acheampong E, Nunnari G, Mukhtar M, Williams KJ, Pomerantz RJ. Human immunodeficiency virus type 1 enters primary human brain microvascular endothelial cells by a mechanism involving cell surface proteoglycans independent of lipid rafts. Journal of Virology. 2003;**77**(22):12140-12151. DOI: 10.1128/jvi.77.22.12140-12151.2003

[13] Bobardt MD, Salmon P, Wang L, Esko JD, Gabuzda D, Fiala M, et al.

Contribution of proteoglycans to human immunodeficiency virus type 1 brain invasion. Journal of Virology. 2004;**78**(12):6567-6584. DOI: 10.1128/JVI.78.12.6567-6584.2004

[14] van Marle G, Gill MJ, Kolodka D, McManus L, Grant T, Church DL. Compartmentalization of the gut viral reservoir in HIV-1-infected patients. Retrovirology. 2007;**4**:87. DOI: 10.1186/1742-4690-4-87

[15] Bednar MM, Sturdevant CB, Tompkins LA, Arrildt KT, Dukhovlinova E, Kincer LP, et al. Compartmentalization, viral evolution, and viral latency of HIV in the CNS. Current HIV/AIDS Reports. 2015;**12**(2):262-271. DOI: 10.1007/s11904-015-0265-9

[16] Walsh JG, Reinke SN, Mamik MK, McKenzie BA, Maingat F, Branton WG, et al. Rapid inflammasome activation in microglia contributes to brain disease in HIV/AIDS. Retrovirology. 2014;**11**:35. DOI: 10.1186/1742-4690-11-35

[17] Uzasci L, Nath A, Cotter R. Oxidative stress and the HIV-infected brain proteome. Journal of Neuroimmune Pharmacology. 2013;**8**(5):1167-1180. DOI: 10.1007/s11481-013-9444-x

[18] Aljawai Y, Richards MH, Seaton MS, Narasipura SD, Al-Harthi L. β-catenin/TCF-4 signaling regulates susceptibility of macrophages and resistance of monocytes to HIV-1 productive infection. Current HIV Research. 2014;**12**(3):164-173. DOI: 10.2174/1570162x12666140526122249

[19] Castellano P, Prevedel L, Eugenin EA. HIV-infected macrophages and microglia that survive acute infection become viral reservoirs by a mechanism involving Bim. Scientific Reports. 2017;**7**(1):12866. DOI: 10.1038/s41598-017-12758-w

[20] Alvarez-Carbonell D, Ye F, Ramanath N, Garcia-Mesa Y, Knapp PE, Hauser KF, et al. Cross-talk between microglia and neurons regulates HIV latency. PLoS Pathogens. 2019;**15**(12):e1008249. DOI: 10.1371/journal.ppat.1008249

[21] Lutgen V, Narasipura SD, Barbian HJ, Richards M, Wallace J, Razmpour R, et al. HIV infects astrocytes in vivo and egresses from the brain to the periphery. PLoS Pathogens. 2020;**16**(6):e1008381. DOI: 10.1371/journal.ppat.1008381

[22] Yu C, Narasipura SD, Richards MH, Hu XT, Yamamoto B, Al-Harthi L. HIV and drug abuse mediate astrocyte senescence in a β-catenin-dependent manner leading to neuronal toxicity. Aging Cell. 2017;**16**(5):956-965. DOI: 10.1111/acel.12593

[23] Schneider M, Tigges B, Meggendorfer M, Helfer M, Ziegenhain C, Brack-Werner R. A new model for post-integration latency in macroglial cells to study HIV-1 reservoirs of the brain. AIDS. 2015;**29**(10):1147-1159. DOI: 10.1097/QAD.0000000000000691

[24] Sturdevant CB, Joseph SB, Schnell G, Price RW, Swanstrom R, Spudich S. Compartmentalized replication of R5 T cell-tropic HIV-1 in the central nervous system early in the course of infection. PLoS Pathogens. 2015;**11**(3):e1004720. DOI: 10.1371/journal.ppat.1004720

[25] Chauhan A, Khandkar M. Endocytosis of human immunodeficiency virus 1 (HIV-1) in astrocytes: A fiery path to its destination. Microbial Pathogenesis. 2015;**78**:1-6. DOI: 10.1016/j.micpath.2014.11.003

[26] Alexaki A, Liu Y, Wigdahl B. Cellular reservoirs of HIV-1 and their role in viral persistence. Current HIV Research. 2008;**6**(5):388-400. DOI: 10.2174/157016208785861195

[27] Anochie PI, Afocha E, Onyeneke EC, Onyeozirila AC, Okoihue A, Ogu AC. Evaluation of the therapeutic efficacy of antiretroviral drugs used in the clinical management of HIV/AIDS infection. Journal of HIV for Clinical and Scientific Research. 2015;**2**(1):023-029. DOI: 10.17352/2455-3786.000010

[28] Arendt G, von Giesen HJ. Antiretroviral therapy regimens for neuro-AIDS. Current Drug Targets Infectious Disorders. 2002;**2**(3):187-192. DOI: 10.2174/1568005023342425

[29] Kranick SM, Nath A. Neurologic complications of HIV-1 infection and its treatment in the era of antiretroviral therapy. Continuum (Minneapolis Minnesota). 2012;**18**(6):1319-1337. DOI: 10.1212/01.CON.0000423849.24900.ec

[30] Letendre S, Marquie-Beck J, Capparelli E, Best B, Clifford D, Collier AC, et al. Validation of the CNS penetration-effectiveness rank for quantifying antiretroviral penetration into the central nervous system. Archives of Neurology. 2008;**65**(1):65-70. DOI: 10.1001/archneurol.2007.31

[31] Osborne O, Peyravian N, Nair M, Daunert S, Toborek M. The paradox of HIV blood-brain barrier penetrance and antiretroviral drug delivery deficiencies. Trends in Neurosciences. 2020;**43**(9):695-708. DOI: 10.1016/j.tins.2020.06.007

[32] Hellmuth J, Valcour V, Spudich S. CNS reservoirs for HIV: Implications for eradication. Journal of Virus Eradication. 2015;**1**(2):67-71. DOI: 10.1016/S2055-6640(20)30489-1

[33] Wang J, Li M, Li J, Deng R. Differences in drug resistance of HIV-1 genotypes in CSF and plasma and analysis of related factors. Virulence. 2023;**14**(1):2171632. DOI: 10.1080/21505594.2023.2171632

[34] Siddiqui A, He C, Lee G, Figueroa A, Slaughter A, Robinson-Papp J. Neuropathogenesis of HIV and emerging therapeutic targets. Expert Opinion on Therapeutic Targets. 2022;**26**(7):603-615. DOI: 10.1080/14728222.2022.2100253

[35] Kelly SH, Nightingale S, Gupta RK, Collier DA. HIV cerebrospinal fluid escape: Interventions for the management, current evidence and future perspectives. Tropical Medicine and Infectious Disease. 2025;**10**(2):45. DOI: 10.3390/tropicalmed10020045

[36] Varghese NM, Senthil V, Saxena SK. Nanocarriers for brain-specific delivery of anti-retroviral drugs: Challenges and achievements. Journal of Drug Targeting. 2018;**26**(3):195-207. DOI: 10.1080/1061186X.2017.1374389

[37] Nowacek A, Gendelman HE. NanoART, neuroAIDS and CNS drug delivery. Nanomedicine (London). 2009;**4**(5):557-574. DOI: 10.2217/nnm.09.38

[38] Gong Y, Chowdhury P, Nagesh PKB, Rahman MA, Zhi K, Yallapu MM, et al. Novel elvitegravir nanoformulation for drug delivery across the blood-brain barrier to achieve HIV-1 suppression in the CNS macrophages. Scientific Reports. 2020;**10**(1):3835. DOI: 10.1038/s41598-020-60684-1

[39] Kumar S, Maurya VK, Dandu HR, Bhatt ML, Saxena SK. Global perspective of novel therapeutic strategies for the management of NeuroAIDS. Biomolecular Concepts. 2018;**9**(1):33-42. DOI: 10.1515/bmc-2018-0005

[40] Mamo T, Moseman EA, Kolishetti N, Salvador-Morales C, Shi J, Kuritzkes DR, et al. Emerging nanotechnology approaches for HIV/AIDS treatment and prevention. Nanomedicine (London). 2010;**5**(2):269-285. DOI: 10.2217/nnm.10.1

[41] Kelly SH, Nightingale S, Gupta RK, Collier DA. HIV cerebrospinal fluid escape: Interventions for the management, current evidence and future perspectives. Tropical Medicine and Infectious Disease. 2025;**10**(2):45. DOI: 10.3390/tropicalmed10020045

[42] McGuire JL, Barrett JS, Vezina HE, Spitsin S, Douglas SD. Adjuvant therapies for HIV-associated neurocognitive disorders. Annals of Clinical Translational Neurology. 2014;**1**(11):938-952. DOI: 10.1002/acn3.131

[43] Klinnert S, Schenkel CD, Freitag PC, Günthard HF, Plückthun A, Metzner KJ. Targeted shock-and-kill HIV-1 gene therapy approach combining CRISPR activation, suicide gene tBid and retargeted adenovirus delivery. Gene Therapy. 2024;**31**(3-4):74-84. DOI: 10.1038/s41434-023-00413-1

[44] Alum EU, Uti DE, Ugwu OP, Alum BN. Toward a cure - Advancing HIV/AIDs treatment modalities beyond antiretroviral therapy: A review. Medicine (Baltimore). 2024;**103**(27):e38768. DOI: 10.1097/MD.0000000000038768

[45] Zhang W, Ruan L. Recent advances in poor HIV immune reconstitution: What will the future look like? Frontiers in Microbiology. 2023;**14**:1236460. DOI: 10.3389/fmicb.2023.1236460

Chapter 2

The Evolution of HIV-1 Drug Resistance and Genetic Variability under HAART Pressure

Bukhari ISah Shuaib, Omosigho Omoruyi Pius and Usman Aliyu Dutsinma

Abstract

The evolution of HIV-1 drug resistance and genetic variability under Highly Active Antiretroviral Therapy (HAART) pressure has been a critical focus of research since the therapy's introduction. HAART, comprising a combination of antiretroviral drugs, revolutionized HIV treatment by reducing viral replication and improving patient outcomes. However, the high mutation rate of HIV-1 facilitates the emergence of drug-resistant variants, particularly under suboptimal drug adherence or incomplete viral suppression. Drug resistance mutations (DRMs) develop in key viral proteins, leading to reduced drug efficacy. Concurrently, the virus exhibits significant genetic variability, driven by recombination and replication errors, further complicating treatment. This review discusses the mechanisms of resistance evolution, the role of genetic variability in resistance development, and how specific drug classes (protease inhibitors, reverse transcriptase inhibitors, integrase strand transfer inhibitors) shape resistance patterns. A comprehensive understanding of the interplay between HAART pressure, resistance, and viral diversity is essential for optimizing therapeutic strategies and developing novel antiretroviral drugs.

Keywords: HIV-1, drug resistance, genetic variability, HAART, therapy

1. Introduction

Human immunodeficiency virus type 1 (HIV-1) remains one of the most significant global health challenges, despite remarkable advancements in treatment and prevention strategies [1]. The discovery of Highly Active Antiretroviral Therapy (HAART) in the mid-1990s marked a turning point in the management of HIV-1, transforming what was once a fatal disease into a manageable chronic condition for millions of individuals worldwide. HAART involves a combination of antiretroviral drugs that target multiple stages of the HIV replication cycle, reducing the viral load to undetectable levels in many patients. By suppressing viral replication, HAART effectively slows the progression of HIV to Acquired Immunodeficiency Syndrome (AIDS) and reduces the risk of transmission [2].

However, even with these significant advances, HIV-1 continues to present formidable challenges due to its high genetic variability and propensity to develop drug resistance. The virus's rapid replication cycle and lack of proofreading mechanisms during reverse transcription lead to frequent mutations in its genome. Under the selective pressure exerted by antiretroviral drugs, particularly during HAART, resistant variants of HIV-1 can emerge and proliferate. Drug resistance is a major concern in the long-term management of HIV-1 infection, as it can compromise the efficacy of treatment, limit future therapeutic options, and increase the likelihood of treatment failure [3].

HIV-1's genetic variability is one of the primary reasons for its persistence and the challenges in managing the infection. HIV-1 belongs to the family of retroviruses and is characterized by its reverse transcription process, in which viral RNA is transcribed into DNA. This process is carried out by the viral enzyme reverse transcriptase, which lacks proofreading capabilities, leading to a high mutation rate. As a result, the virus generates a diverse population of viral variants, known as quasi-species, within a single infected individual. This genetic diversity allows HIV-1 to adapt rapidly to different selective pressures, including immune responses and antiretroviral drugs [4, 5].

HIV-1 is classified into four major groups: M (major), N (non-M, non-O), O (outlier), and P. Group M are responsible for the global pandemic and are further divided into subtypes (A through K) and circulating recombinant forms (CRFs). These subtypes exhibit genetic differences that can influence their replication rates, transmission dynamics, and susceptibility to antiretroviral drugs. In regions where multiple subtypes co-circulate, recombination between different viral strains further increases the genetic diversity of HIV-1. This genetic variability complicates treatment efforts, as different subtypes may respond differently to specific drugs or develop resistance through distinct pathways [5].

Despite the effectiveness of HAART in controlling HIV-1 replication, the development of drug-resistant strains remains a major concern for long-term treatment success. Drug resistance arises when mutations in the HIV genome reduce the efficacy of antiretroviral drugs, allowing the virus to continue replicating in the presence of therapy [6, 7]. These mutations may pre-exist in the viral quasi-species before treatment or emerge during therapy, particularly when viral replication is not fully suppressed. The selective pressure exerted by antiretroviral drugs means that only variants capable of evading drug effects will survive and proliferate. Over time, resistant strains may become dominant within the viral population. Several factors contribute to the emergence of drug resistance, including poor adherence to treatment, which allows the virus to replicate intermittently, suboptimal drug concentrations due to improper dosing or drug interactions, and pre-existing resistance in patients infected with resistant strains. Once resistant variants emerge, they can lead to treatment failure, requiring a switch to second-line or salvage therapies. The genetic diversity of HIV-1 further complicates the management of drug resistance, as different subtypes and recombinants may develop resistance through different pathways and respond differently to antiretroviral drugs. This makes continuous monitoring and adaptation of treatment strategies essential for maintaining long-term viral suppression and treatment efficacy [8].

The primary objective of this review is to provide a comprehensive examination of the evolution of HIV-1 drug resistance and genetic variability under HAART pressure. Specifically, the review will:

1. Explore the mechanisms by which HIV-1 develops drug resistance, focusing on the genetic mutations that confer resistance to different classes of antiretroviral drugs.

2. Examine the role of viral genetic diversity in the emergence of drug-resistant strains, including the impact of viral subtypes and recombination on resistance patterns.

3. Assess the clinical implications of drug resistance, including its impact on treatment outcomes, the management of treatment failure, and the development of next-generation therapies.

4. Discuss future directions for overcoming the challenges posed by HIV-1 drug resistance, including the development of new drugs, gene therapy approaches, and potential cure strategies.

2. The HIV-1 epidemic and its global impact

Human immunodeficiency virus type 1 (HIV-1) has been a major public health crisis since its identification in the early 1980s. As of 2023, more than 38 million people worldwide are living with HIV-1, with millions of deaths attributed to AIDS-related illnesses. While the global response has significantly improved through advances in treatment and prevention, HIV-1 remains a leading cause of morbidity and mortality, particularly in sub-Saharan Africa (**Figure 1**), where nearly two-thirds of all HIV-1 cases are concentrated [9, 10].

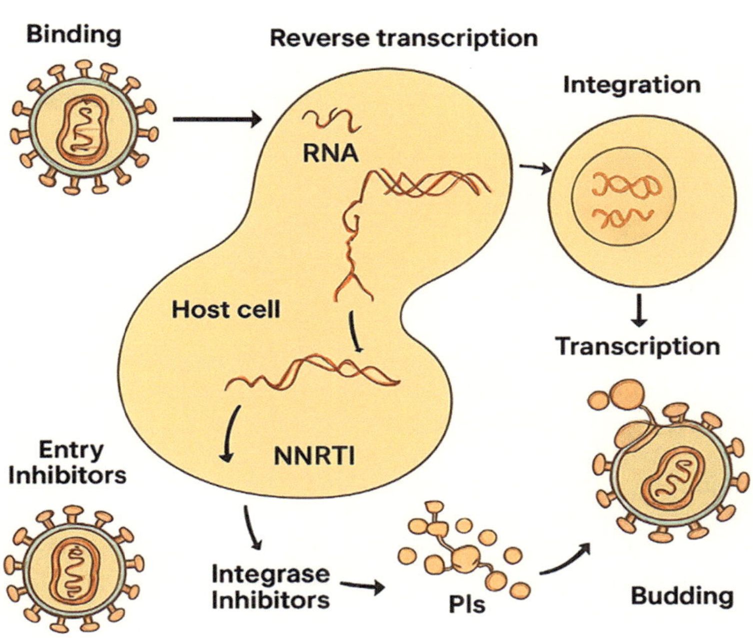

Figure 1.
HIV-1 life cycle and HAART targets (Illustration *showing key steps of the HIV-1 life cycle, such as binding, reverse transcription, integration, transcription, translation, and budding, with drug classes targeting each step).*

Region	Dominant subtype(s)	Estimated cases (Millions)
Sub-Saharan Africa	Subtype C	25
North America	Subtype B	2
Asia	Subtype AE	5
Europe	Subtype B	1.5

Table 1.
Global distribution of HIV-1 subtypes.

HIV-1 is a lentivirus, a member of the retrovirus family, that primarily targets and depletes CD4+ T lymphocytes, critical cells in the human immune system. The depletion of these cells leads to immunosuppression, rendering individuals vulnerable to opportunistic infections and cancers, the hallmark of acquired immunodeficiency syndrome (AIDS). The virus is transmitted through several routes, including unprotected sexual contact, intravenous drug use, mother-to-child transmission during birth or breastfeeding, and blood transfusions. The global spread of HIV-1 is characterized by different patterns of infection, with certain subtypes dominating in specific regions. This geographic variation contributes to the challenges in treatment and management due to differences in viral evolution and resistance as shown in **Table 1** [5, 11].

2.1 HIV-1 life cycle and replication

The life cycle of HIV-1 is essential to comprehend how antiretroviral therapies (ART) and Highly Active Antiretroviral Therapy (HAART) exert their effects on the virus. HIV-1 replicates through a multi-step process that involves entering the host cell, reverse transcription of viral RNA into DNA, integration of viral DNA into the host genome, transcription and translation of viral proteins, assembly of new virions, and budding from the host cell. These steps provide multiple therapeutic targets for antiretroviral drugs as shown in **Figure 1** [12, 13].

1. Binding and fusion: HIV-1 initiates infection by binding to CD4 receptors on the surface of target cells (primarily CD4+ T cells), and co-receptors such as CCR5 or CXCR4. After binding, the viral envelope fuses with the host cell membrane, allowing the viral capsid to enter the cytoplasm.

2. Reverse transcription: Inside the host cell, the viral RNA genome is reverse transcribed into double-stranded DNA by the enzyme reverse transcriptase, a key step targeted by several classes of antiretroviral drugs.

3. Integration: The viral DNA is then transported into the nucleus and integrated into the host cell genome by the viral enzyme integrase. Once integrated, the viral DNA, known as provirus, can remain dormant or be transcribed to produce new viral particles.

4. Transcription and translation: The host cell machinery transcribes the integrated provirus into viral RNA, which is used to produce viral proteins, including structural proteins, enzymes, and components of the viral envelope.

5. Assembly and budding: Newly synthesized viral proteins and RNA assemble at the cell membrane, where they bud off to form new virions. The viral enzyme protease cleaves precursor proteins into their functional forms, a critical step in the maturation of infectious viral particles.

2.1.1 Subtype-specific differences

HIV-1 subtypes show differences in their propensity to develop certain resistance mutations. For instance, subtype B, which predominates in North America and Europe, is more likely to develop the K103N mutation in response to NNRTI therapy, while subtype C, which is more common in sub-Saharan Africa, may be less prone to this mutation but more likely to develop other NNRTI resistance mutations such as Y181C [14, 15]. This subtype variability means that resistance testing and treatment strategies need to be tailored to the specific viral subtype present in a given population.

Subtype-specific differences in drug resistance also have important implications for global HIV treatment efforts, as different regions of the world are dominated by different HIV-1 subtypes. As HAART is scaled up in resource-limited settings, particularly in regions where non-subtype B viruses predominate, understanding the resistance patterns associated with these subtypes is crucial for developing effective treatment guidelines [16, 17].

2.2 The development of HAART: A paradigm shift in HIV treatment

The introduction of HAART in the mid-1990s revolutionized HIV treatment by combining multiple antiretroviral drugs, usually from at least two different drug classes, to suppress viral replication. Prior to HAART, treatment options were limited to single-drug therapies, such as zidovudine (AZT), which provided only temporary suppression of viral replication [6]. Monotherapy quickly led to the emergence of drug-resistant HIV strains, resulting in treatment failure and progression to AIDS. The rationale behind this combination therapy is to target different stages of the HIV life cycle, thereby reducing the likelihood that the virus can escape treatment through single mutations. By dramatically reducing viral replication, HAART not only prolongs the life of HIV-infected individuals but also significantly reduces the risk of transmission, particularly in cases of mother-to-child transmission and among key populations such as men who have sex with men (MSM) and intravenous drug users [8]. HAART changed this dynamic by introducing combination therapy, using multiple drugs from different classes to target various stages of the HIV-1 life cycle. By attacking the virus at several points in its replication process, HAART achieved more durable viral suppression, preventing the rapid development of resistance and allowing for long-term control of the infection [9]. The combination of drugs with the distinct mechanisms of action made it much harder for the virus to develop resistance mutations that would render all the drugs in the regimen ineffective.

HAART typically includes drugs from multiple classes that target different stages of the HIV lifecycle. Nucleoside reverse transcriptase inhibitors (NRTIs) mimic natural nucleosides, causing chain termination and preventing viral replication [11]. Non-nucleoside reverse transcriptase inhibitors (NNRTIs) bind directly to reverse transcriptase, inhibiting its activity and further disrupting viral replication [3]. Protease inhibitors (PIs) inhibit the HIV protease enzyme, preventing the production of functional viral proteins needed to form infectious viral particles. Integrase strand transfer inhibitors (INSTIs) prevent the viral integrase enzyme from integrating HIV DNA into the host genome, blocking a key step in the infection process [6]. Less commonly used drugs, such as entry and fusion inhibitors, block the virus from entering host cells by interfering with viral fusion or receptor interactions. The combination of these drugs from different classes not only enhances viral suppression but also reduces the likelihood of drug resistance emerging through single mutations. This multi-pronged approach has made HAART highly effective in reducing viral load, slowing disease progression, and minimizing transmission risk. However, the success of HAART hinges on strict adherence to the prescribed regimen, as lapses can lead to viral rebound and resistance [18].

2.3 Mechanisms of action of HAART

The success of HAART lies in its multi-faceted approach to viral suppression. Each class of drugs in HAART targets a specific stage of the HIV replication cycle, thereby reducing viral load and limiting the opportunity for the virus to develop resistance. By using multiple drugs simultaneously, HAART ensures that even if the virus develops resistance to one drug, the other drugs in the regimen can continue to suppress viral replication (**Table 2**).

The key drug classes used in HAART are as follows:

1. Nucleoside reverse transcriptase inhibitors (NRTIs): NRTIs, such as zidovudine (AZT), lamivudine (3TC), and tenofovir (TDF), act at the reverse transcription stage or mimic the natural nucleosides that HIV uses to synthesize DNA, preventing the conversion of viral RNA into DNA. This early intervention in the HIV replication cycle is crucial for stopping the virus from integrating into the host cell genome [9].

2. Non-nucleoside reverse transcriptase inhibitors (NNRTIs): NNRTIs, such as efavirenz (EFV) and nevirapine (NVP), bind directly to reverse transcriptase and inhibit its activity. Unlike NRTIs, NNRTIs do not require phosphorylation to become active and bind to a different site on the reverse transcriptase enzyme, resulting in conformational changes that prevent the enzyme from functioning [6].

3. Protease inhibitors (PIs): PIs, such as ritonavir (RTV) and lopinavir (LPV), inhibit the activity of the HIV-1 protease enzyme, which is essential for processing viral proteins into their mature forms. Without functional protease, the virus produces immature, non-infectious virions [5].

Drug class	Mutation example	Effect on drug efficacy
NRTIs	M184V	High resistance to 3TC
NNRTIs	K103N	Resistance to efavirenz
Protease inhibitors	L90M	Cross-resistance to PIs
Integrase inhibitors	Q148H	Resistance to raltegravir

Table 2.
Key resistance mutations by drug class.

4. Integrase strand transfer inhibitors (INSTIs): INSTIs, such as raltegravir (RAL) and dolutegravir (DTG), target the integrase enzyme, which HIV-1 uses to integrate its DNA into the host cell genome. By blocking this step, INSTIs prevent the establishment of productive infection [9].

5. Entry and fusion inhibitors: These less commonly used drugs, such as maraviroc (MVC) and enfuvirtide (T-20), block the initial steps of HIV entry into the host cell by targeting the interaction between the virus and the CD4 receptor or the fusion of the viral envelope with the host cell membrane [11].

2.4 The benefits and challenges of HAART

2.4.1 Benefits of HAART

HAART has revolutionized the treatment of HIV-1, transforming the infection from a terminal illness into a manageable chronic disease for most patients. Some of the major benefits of HAART include:

1. Prolonged life expectancy: HAART has been instrumental in extending the life expectancy of HIV-infected individuals. Patients who adhere to HAART can expect near-normal life spans, provided they initiate treatment early and maintain good viral suppression [19].

2. Reduction in AIDS-related morbidity and mortality: Before HAART, most individuals infected with HIV-1 eventually progressed to AIDS, characterized by opportunistic infections, cancers, and a high mortality rate. HAART significantly reduces the risk of these complications by preserving immune function and suppressing viral replication [12].

3. Reduction in HIV transmission: HAART not only benefits the individual but also plays a critical role in public health by reducing the risk of HIV transmission. Studies have shown that individuals with undetectable viral loads are much less likely to transmit the virus to sexual partners, leading to the "Undetectable = Untransmittable" (U=U) campaign [7].

4. Prevention of mother-to-child transmission: HAART has been highly effective in preventing the transmission of HIV-1 from pregnant women to their infants, especially when initiated early in pregnancy and continued through breastfeeding [5].

2.4.2 Challenges of HAART

While HAART has greatly improved the prognosis for people living with HIV, it is not without challenges [7, 11, 15]:

1. Drug resistance: One of the most significant challenges is the emergence of drug-resistant HIV-1 strains. Poor adherence to HAART, suboptimal drug levels, or pre-existing resistance mutations can lead to treatment failure and the need for second-line or salvage therapies.

2. Adherence: Maintaining strict adherence to HAART is essential for achieving and sustaining viral suppression

3. Non-adherence can result in viral rebound, resistance development, and treatment failure. Adherence can be influenced by factors such as pill burden, side effects, and psychosocial factors.

4. Side effects and toxicity: Although newer antiretroviral drugs are generally safer and better tolerated than earlier generations, side effects remain a concern. Common side effects include gastrointestinal disturbances, liver toxicity, lipid abnormalities, and cardiovascular risks. Long-term use of HAART can also lead to complications such as bone density loss and kidney damage.

5. Cost and accessibility: The cost of HAART remains a barrier, especially in resource-limited settings. While global initiatives have improved access to antiretroviral therapy, disparities still exist in many regions, and ensuring sustained access to treatment is a challenge.

2.5 Evolution of HAART over time

Since its inception, HAART has evolved considerably, with the improvements in drug formulations, regimens, and delivery systems. Early HAART regimens were often complex, requiring multiple pills taken several times a day, with significant side effects. However, newer regimens are simpler, often consisting of single-tablet formulations taken once daily, making adherence easier and improving patient outcomes [5, 19].

Furthermore, the development of more potent and better-tolerated drugs, particularly integrase inhibitors, has significantly improved the effectiveness of HAART. Current guidelines recommend starting treatment as soon as possible after diagnosis, regardless of CD4 count, a practice known as "treat all" or "universal treatment [3]."

2.6 Mechanisms of HIV-1 drug resistance

One of the most significant challenges in the long-term management of HIV-1 infection is the development of drug resistance, which can compromise the effectiveness of antiretroviral therapy (ART) and lead to treatment failure. The mechanisms of HIV-1 drug resistance are rooted in the virus's ability to rapidly mutate and evolve under the selective pressure exerted by antiretroviral drugs, particularly in the context of highly active antiretroviral therapy (HAART). Drug resistance arises when the virus acquires mutations in its genome that reduce the efficacy of one or more drugs, allowing the virus to continue replicating even in the presence of therapy [6, 20].

HIV-1's high mutation rate, coupled with the selective pressure of HAART, creates an environment where drug-resistant variants can emerge and proliferate. Understanding the mechanisms of drug resistance is critical for designing effective treatment strategies, preventing the spread of resistant strains, and developing new therapies that can overcome resistance [12, 17].

2.6.1 Mutation and selective pressure

2.6.1.1 HIV-1's high mutation rate

HIV-1 is characterized by an exceptionally high mutation rate, which is a key factor in the development of drug resistance. The virus replicates through a process called reverse transcription, where its RNA genome is transcribed into DNA by the viral enzyme reverse transcriptase. Unlike many other enzymes, reverse transcriptase lacks proofreading capabilities, meaning it does not correct errors that occur during the transcription process. As a result, HIV-1 accumulates mutations at a rate of approximately 1 mutation per 10,000 nucleotides per replication cycle. Given that the HIV-1 genome is about 9700 nucleotides long, this means that on average, every newly produced virion contains at least one mutation [21, 22].

In addition to reverse transcriptase's intrinsic error rate, HIV-1 undergoes rapid replication, with billions of virions produced daily in an infected individual. This high replication rate, combined with the lack of proofreading, results in a highly diverse viral population known as a "quasispecies." Within this quasispecies, different variants may carry mutations that confer varying levels of fitness, including resistance to antiretroviral drugs [3, 6, 10].

2.6.1.2 Selective pressure from antiretroviral drugs

Selective pressure is the process by which certain environmental factors, such as antiretroviral drugs, favor the survival and replication of specific viral variants that possess advantageous mutations. In the context of HIV-1 infection, the introduction of HAART creates a strong selective pressure, as only those variants that can evade the inhibitory effects of the drugs will continue to replicate. This pressure can lead to the emergence and eventual dominance of drug-resistant strains, especially if viral replication is not fully suppressed by the treatment regimen [9, 13].

The development of drug resistance is typically a stepwise process. Initially, the viral population is composed of both drug-sensitive and drug-resistant variants. When HAART is introduced, the drugs effectively suppress the replication of drug-sensitive variants. However, if the drugs fail to completely inhibit viral replication (due to poor adherence, suboptimal drug levels, or pre-existing low-frequency resistance mutations), drug-resistant variants may continue to replicate and gradually become the dominant strain [6, 12, 15].

There are several factors that contribute to the selective pressure exerted by antiretroviral drugs:

1. *Drug potency and genetic barrier to resistance:* Some antiretroviral drugs are more potent than others, meaning they require fewer mutations to lose effectiveness. Drugs with a low genetic barrier to resistance, such as non-nucleoside reverse transcriptase inhibitors (NNRTIs), may be rendered ineffective by a single mutation in the viral genome. In contrast, drugs with a high genetic barrier to resistance, such as protease inhibitors (PIs) and integrase strand transfer inhibitors (INSTIs), require multiple mutations before the virus becomes resistant [21].

2. *Adherence to treatment:* Strict adherence to HAART is crucial for maintaining viral suppression. Incomplete or inconsistent adherence allows the virus to replicate intermittently, increasing the likelihood that resistant variants will emerge. Even brief lapses in adherence can result in a rapid increase in viral load, providing opportunities for the virus to mutate and develop resistance [22].

3. *Drug levels and pharmacokinetics:* Suboptimal drug concentrations, whether due to poor absorption, drug interactions, or incorrect dosing, can lead to incomplete

suppression of viral replication. In such cases, the virus may continue replicating in the presence of sub-therapeutic drug levels, increasing the risk of resistance mutations [19].

4. *Viral fitness:* Some drug-resistant mutations come at a cost to viral fitness, meaning the resistant strains may replicate less efficiently than wild-type, drug-sensitive strains. However, under strong selective pressure from antiretroviral drugs, even less fit resistant variants can outcompete sensitive strains. Over time, compensatory mutations may restore the fitness of the resistant strains, allowing them to replicate efficiently despite the presence of resistance mutations [17].

2.6.2 Types of resistance mutations

HIV-1 drug resistance mutations can be classified into two broad categories: primary mutations and secondary (compensatory) mutations [2].

Primary resistance mutations: These mutations directly reduce the effectiveness of antiretroviral drugs by altering the target site of the drug or interfering with the drug's mechanism of action. For example, mutations in the reverse transcriptase gene can reduce the binding affinity of NRTIs and NNRTIs, while mutations in the protease gene can affect the binding of protease inhibitors. Primary mutations are often the first to emerge under drug pressure and are typically associated with high-level resistance to a specific drug [7].

Secondary (compensatory) mutations: While primary mutations are necessary for the development of drug resistance, they often reduce the overall fitness of the virus, making it less efficient at replicating. Secondary mutations, also known as compensatory mutations, help restore viral fitness by compensating for the deleterious effects of the primary mutations. These mutations may not directly confer drug resistance, but they enhance the replication capacity of the resistant virus, allowing it to persist and proliferate in the presence of antiretroviral therapy [10].

Together, primary and secondary mutations form a complex network of resistance that can significantly reduce the effectiveness of HAART. The accumulation of multiple mutations, particularly in combination with compensatory mutations, can lead to cross-resistance, where the virus becomes resistant to several drugs within the same class, or even across different classes of antiretroviral drugs [2, 4].

2.6.2.1 Examples of key resistance mutations

Different classes of antiretroviral drugs are associated with specific resistance mutations, depending on their mechanism of action and the viral enzymes they target. Some key examples of resistance mutations include the following:

1. *Nucleoside reverse transcriptase inhibitors (NRTIs):* Resistance to NRTIs often involves mutations in the reverse transcriptase enzyme that affect the incorporation of the drug into the viral DNA chain [8]. Common mutations include the following:

   a. *M184V/I:* This mutation occurs in the reverse transcriptase gene and confers high-level resistance to lamivudine (3TC) and emtricitabine (FTC). However, it also reduces viral fitness and increases susceptibility to certain other NRTIs, such as zidovudine (AZT) [12].

b. *K65R:* This mutation confers resistance to tenofovir (TDF) and other NRTIs by reducing the efficiency of drug incorporation into the viral DNA [14].

2. *Non-nucleoside reverse transcriptase inhibitors (NNRTIs):* NNRTI resistance typically involves mutations in the reverse transcriptase gene that affect the binding of the drug to its allosteric site [23]. Common mutations include the following:

   a. *K103N:* This mutation confers high-level resistance to efavirenz (EFV) and nevirapine (NVP) by preventing the drug from binding to reverse transcriptase [11].

   b. *Y181C:* This mutation reduces susceptibility to several NNRTIs, including nevirapine and efavirenz, by altering the drug-binding site on reverse transcriptase [12].

3. *Protease inhibitors (PIs):* Resistance to PIs arises from mutations in the protease enzyme that reduce the binding of the drug while preserving the enzyme's ability to cleave viral proteins [18]. Common mutations include the following:

   a. *D30N:* This mutation confers resistance to nelfinavir (NFV) by altering the protease enzyme, preventing the drug from binding effectively [12].

   b. *L90M:* This mutation is associated with resistance to multiple PIs, including lopinavir (LPV) and ritonavir (RTV), by affecting the protease active site [4].

4. *Integrase strand transfer inhibitors (INSTIs):* Resistance to INSTIs involves mutations in the integrase enzyme that reduce the drug's ability to block viral DNA integration [11]. Common mutations include the following:

   a. *N155H:* This mutation confers resistance to early-generation INSTIs, such as raltegravir (RAL) and elvitegravir (EVG), by altering the integrase enzyme's active site [5].

   b. *Q148H/K/R:* These mutations are associated with high-level resistance to INSTIs and can lead to cross-resistance among drugs in this class [24].

2.6.3 Clinical implications of drug resistance

The development of drug resistance has significant clinical implications for the management of HIV-1 infection. Drug-resistant strains can lead to treatment failure, requiring patients to switch to second-line or third-line therapies, which are often more expensive and may have a higher pill burden or more side effects. Additionally, once resistance mutations have emerged, they may persist in the viral reservoir even if the patient switches to a different regimen, limiting future treatment options [6, 10, 15].

Moreover, the transmission of drug-resistant HIV-1 strains is a growing concern, particularly in regions with the limited access to resistance testing and newer antiretroviral drugs. Transmitted drug resistance (TDR) occurs when an individual is infected with a strain of HIV-1 that already carries resistance mutations, which can complicate treatment from the outset [4, 25]. HIV-1's high mutation rate and the selective pressure exerted by HAART create an environment where drug-resistant variants can emerge and proliferate [21, 23].

2.7 Genetic variability of HIV-1 under HAART pressure

HIV-1 exhibits extraordinary genetic variability, driven by its high mutation rate, rapid replication cycle, and the absence of error-correction mechanisms during reverse transcription. This genetic diversity complicates the management of HIV-1 infection, particularly in the context of highly active antiretroviral therapy (HAART) [21]. The virus's ability to mutate and evolve under drug pressure not only leads to the emergence of drug-resistant strains but also results in a dynamic population of closely related viral variants, collectively referred to as viral quasi-species [12]. These quasi-species form the genetic foundation that enables HIV-1 to adapt to various selective pressures, including the immune response and antiretroviral drugs [12, 26].

2.7.1 The role of viral quasi-species

2.7.1.1 Defining viral quasi-species

The concept of viral quasi-species refers to the highly heterogeneous population of genetically related variants within an individual infected with HIV-1 [7, 9, 27]. These variants arise due to the error-prone replication of the virus, particularly during reverse transcription, where the reverse transcriptase enzyme introduces frequent mutations (**Figure 2**). Because HIV-1 lacks a proofreading mechanism, these mutations accumulate rapidly, resulting in a swarm of viral variants that coexist within the same host. Each variant within the quasi-species may differ by one or more mutations,

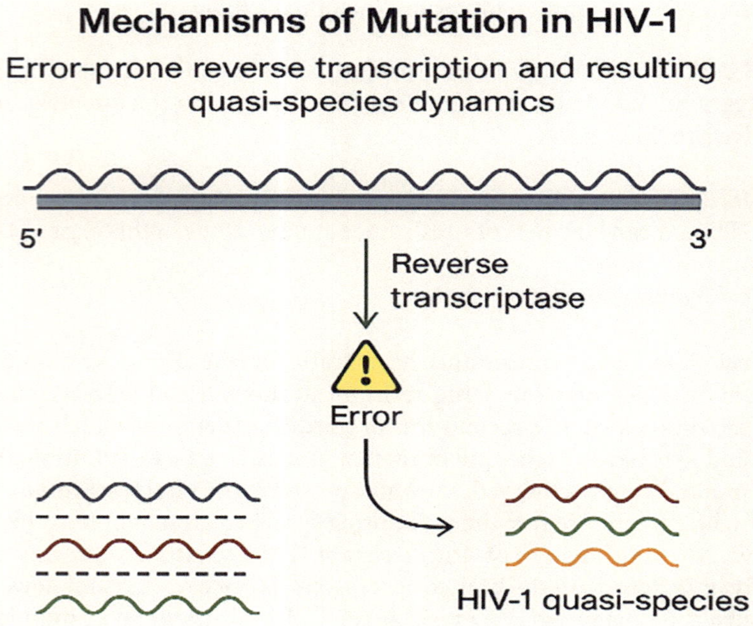

Figure 2.
Mechanisms of mutation in HIV-1 (Diagram illustrating the error-prone reverse transcription process and the resulting quasi-species dynamics).

creating a complex, dynamic population of viruses that constantly evolve under selective pressures such as the host immune system and antiretroviral therapy [28, 29].

The quasi-species model is distinct from the clonal evolution of many other pathogens, where a single dominant strain may predominate. In HIV-1 infection, the viral population is better understood as a "cloud" of related but distinct variants that continuously interact, compete, and evolve. These quasi-species provide a reservoir of genetic diversity that allows the virus to adapt quickly to environmental changes, such as the introduction of HAART. The genetic diversity inherent in quasi-species contributes to the rapid development of drug resistance and immune escape [5, 7, 12].

2.7.1.2 Generation of quasi-species in HIV-1

Several factors contribute to the generation and maintenance of viral quasi-species in HIV-1:

1. High mutation rate: HIV-1 reverse transcriptase introduces mutations at a high frequency during the reverse transcription process, with an estimated error rate of 1 in 10,000 nucleotides per replication cycle. Given the virus's relatively short genome (approximately 9.7 kilobases) and rapid replication rate, each new virion is likely to carry at least one mutation compared to its parent virus [8, 13].

2. Rapid replication cycle: HIV-1 has an extremely fast replication cycle, with millions to billions of new virions produced daily in an infected individual. This rapid turnover of viral particles ensures that the viral population remains genetically diverse and dynamic, with new mutations constantly introduced into the quasi-species pool [9, 22].

3. Lack of proofreading mechanisms: Unlike many other viruses or host DNA replication processes, HIV-1 lacks a proofreading mechanism in its reverse transcriptase enzyme. This absence of error correction allows mutations to persist and accumulate during each cycle of replication, increasing the genetic diversity of the viral population [18, 20, 25].

4. Recombination: HIV-1 can undergo genetic recombination when two or more viral genomes are present in the same host cell. If a single cell is infected with multiple HIV-1 virions, segments of their genomes can be exchanged during reverse transcription, producing recombinant viruses. Recombination enhances the genetic diversity of the viral quasi-species and can lead to the emergence of new variants with combinations of drug resistance mutations [21, 27, 29].

2.7.1.3 The impact of HAART on viral quasi-species

The introduction of HAART exerts strong selective pressure on the HIV-1 population, significantly influencing the composition of the quasi-species. HAART's primary goal is to suppress viral replication to undetectable levels, reducing the opportunity for new variants to emerge. However, incomplete suppression or inconsistent adherence to therapy can allow replication to continue in the presence of antiretroviral drugs, selecting for drug-resistant variants within the quasi-species [16, 20, 26].

Selection of drug-resistant variants: HAART creates an environment where drug-sensitive variants are suppressed, while pre-existing or newly generated drug-resistant variants within the quasi-species may continue to replicate. These resistant variants can quickly become the dominant strain in the viral population if selective pressure from HAART persists, leading to the treatment failure. The presence of quasi-species increases the likelihood that resistant variants are present before therapy is initiated, especially in individuals with a long history of untreated infection or exposure to suboptimal therapies [21, 23, 27].

Shifts in quasi-species composition: Under HAART pressure, the composition of the viral quasi-species shifts over time. Initially, the viral population may be dominated by drug-sensitive variants, but as treatment progresses and resistance mutations accumulate, drug-resistant variants can emerge and become the predominant strains. This shift is influenced by factors such as the potency of the drugs, adherence to therapy, and the genetic barrier to resistance. In some cases, multiple drug-resistant variants may coexist within the quasi-species, each with different resistance mutations targeting specific drugs in the HAART regimen [21, 27, 30].

Minority variants and resistance development: One of the key features of HIV-1 quasi-species is the presence of minority variants—genetically distinct subpopulations that exist at low frequencies within the viral population. These minority variants can carry drug resistance mutations, even if they are not the dominant strain at the time of diagnosis or treatment initiation. Under the selective pressure of HAART, these minority variants can expand and become dominant, leading to treatment failure. The detection of minority variants is challenging with the standard diagnostic techniques, which typically only identify the dominant strain, but their presence is a significant factor in the emergence of drug resistance [21, 27, 30].

2.7.1.4 Role of quasi-species in drug resistance evolution

The dynamic nature of HIV-1 quasi-species plays a critical role in the evolution of drug resistance under HAART pressure. Several mechanisms contribute to this process:

1. *Pre-existing resistance mutations:* Within the quasi-species, there may be variants that already carry mutations conferring resistance to specific antiretroviral drugs, even before therapy is initiated. These pre-existing resistance mutations may have arisen spontaneously through the high mutation rate or recombination events. When HAART is introduced, these pre-existing resistant variants can be selected for and expand, leading to treatment failure [13, 19].

2. *De novo mutations:* Even if the quasi-species initially lacks significant resistance mutations, the ongoing replication of HIV-1 in the presence of HAART increases the likelihood that new mutations will arise that confer resistance to one or more drugs in the regimen. These *de novo* mutations may emerge in a stepwise fashion, with one mutation conferring partial resistance, followed by additional mutations that lead to high-level resistance [30, 31].

3. *Compensatory mutations:* In some cases, resistance mutations can reduce the fitness of the virus, making it less efficient at replicating. However, the quasi-species model allows for the accumulation of compensatory mutations, which restores viral fitness while maintaining drug resistance. These compensatory

mutations may arise in other parts of the viral genome or in the same gene as the resistance mutations [26, 28].

4. *Cross-resistance:* As resistance mutations accumulate within the quasi-species, the virus may develop cross-resistance to multiple drugs within the same class or across different classes. For example, mutations that confer resistance to one protease inhibitor may also reduce susceptibility to other protease inhibitors. The quasi-species model facilitates the accumulation of mutations that lead to broad resistance profiles, complicating treatment options [4, 6, 29].

5. *Recombination and resistance evolution:* Recombination between different viral variants within the quasi-species can create new viral genomes that combine resistance mutations from multiple parent viruses. This process can lead to the emergence of highly resistant recombinant viruses that are more difficult to treat. Recombination can also accelerate the evolution of resistance by bringing together mutations that might not have arisen through point mutations alone [25, 30].

2.7.1.5 Clinical implications of quasi-species in HAART

The genetic variability of HIV-1 and the quasi-species model have several important clinical implications for the management of HIV-1 infection under HAART pressure:

1. *Challenges in resistance testing:* Standard genotypic and phenotypic resistance testing typically detects the dominant viral strain, which may not fully represent the diversity of the quasi-species. Minority variants with resistance mutations may go undetected, leading to an underestimation of the true level of drug resistance. This limitation can result in suboptimal treatment choices, as clinicians may select drugs that appear effective based on the dominant strain but are ineffective against minority resistant variants [12, 32].

2. *Treatment failure and resistance:* The presence of drug-resistant variants within the quasi-species increases the risk of treatment failure, particularly if adherence to HAART is suboptimal or if drug levels are insufficient to fully suppress viral replication. Incomplete suppression allows resistant variants to emerge and expand, ultimately leading to virological failure [29, 31].

3. *Therapeutic strategies:* Understanding the role of quasi-species in drug resistance evolution underscores the importance of selecting potent, high-genetic-barrier regimens that can suppress a broad range of viral variants. Early and aggressive treatment is crucial to reducing the genetic diversity of the viral population and preventing the emergence of resistance. Additionally, the use of resistance testing and therapeutic drug monitoring can help tailor treatment to the specific quasi-species present in each patient [12, 32].

4. *Future directions:* Advances in deep sequencing technologies and the development of more sensitive diagnostic tools may improve the detection of minority variants within the quasi-species, allowing for more personalized treatment strategies. These technologies can provide a more comprehensive view of the viral

population, enabling clinicians to anticipate resistance development and adjust therapy accordingly [22, 26].

2.8 Clinical implications of HIV-1 drug resistance and genetic variability

The evolution of HIV-1 drug resistance and the genetic variability of the virus present significant challenges for the clinical management of HIV-1 infection. HIV-1's high mutation rate, coupled with the selective pressure from highly active antiretroviral therapy (HAART), leads to the emergence of resistant strains that can compromise treatment efficacy [33]. Drug resistance and viral genetic diversity can influence treatment outcomes, affect long-term viral suppression, and limit the effectiveness of available antiretroviral drugs [12]. The clinical implications of HIV-1 drug resistance extend beyond individual patient care, impacting public health strategies for controlling the spread of resistant strains. These clinical implications are essential for optimizing treatment strategies, tailoring therapy to individual patients, and mitigating the broader consequences of drug resistance [31, 33].

2.8.1 Impact on treatment outcomes

The development of drug resistance and the genetic diversity of HIV-1 under HAART pressure significantly impact treatment outcomes. These factors can lead to virological failure, limit future treatment options, and increase the likelihood of disease progression [12, 31].

2.8.1.1 Virological failure and resistance development

One of the most direct clinical consequences of HIV-1 drug resistance is virological failure (**Figure 3**), which occurs when antiretroviral therapy is unable to achieve or maintain viral suppression. Virological failure is typically defined as a rebound in plasma HIV-1 RNA levels despite ongoing therapy, often due to the emergence of drug-resistant strains within the viral population. Resistance mutations that arise in response to HAART reduce the efficacy of the drugs, allowing the virus to continue replicating in the presence of therapy [31, 34].

Several factors contribute to the development of drug resistance and subsequent virological failure:

Suboptimal drug adherence: Adherence to HAART is critical for achieving and maintaining viral suppression. Inconsistent or incomplete adherence allows viral replication to continue in the presence of sub-therapeutic drug levels, increasing the likelihood that resistance mutations will emerge. Poor adherence is one of the most common causes of treatment failure and the development of resistance [12, 24, 30].

Low genetic barrier to resistance: Some antiretroviral drugs, such as non-nucleoside reverse transcriptase inhibitors (NNRTIs), have a low genetic barrier to resistance, meaning that only one or two mutations are needed for the virus to become resistant. The rapid acquisition of these mutations can lead to virological failure, especially if the patient is not fully adherent to therapy [12, 35].

Pre-existing resistance mutations: In some cases, drug-resistant variants may already be present within the viral population before therapy is initiated. These pre-existing mutations may have arisen due to previous exposure to antiretroviral drugs or transmitted drug resistance (TDR). If these variants are not detected through resistance testing, they can lead to early treatment failure as resistant strains expand under drug pressure.

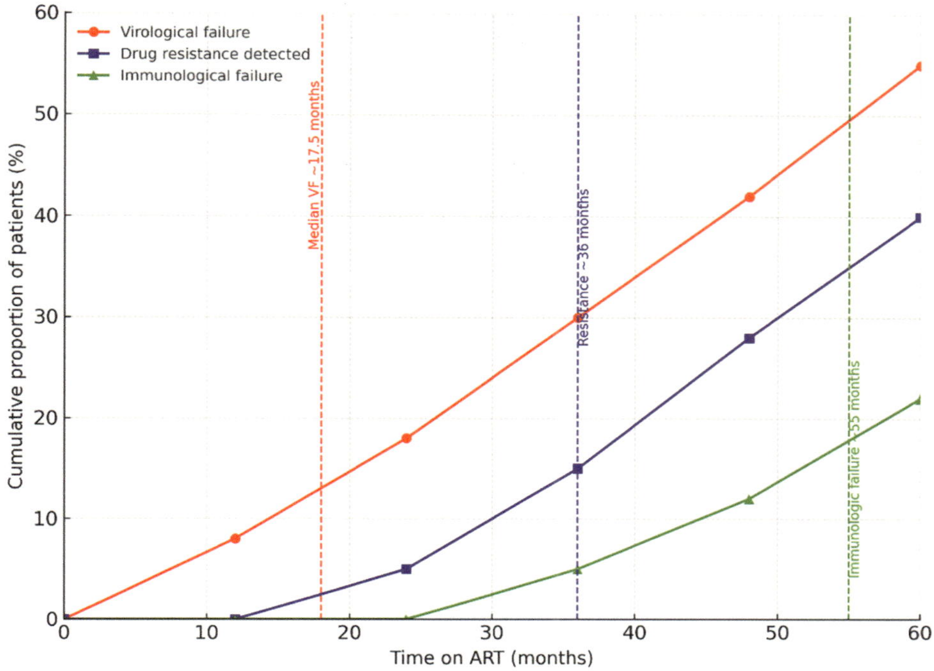

Figure 3.
Virological failure in HAART (graph showing the rates of virological failure over time due to resistance development.)

Virological failure is a major concern because it necessitates changes to the treatment regimen. Switching to second-line or third-line therapies often involves more complex drug combinations, higher pill burdens, and an increased risk of side effects. Moreover, the pool of effective drugs becomes smaller with each episode of virological failure, as the virus accumulates additional resistance mutations [23, 29, 32].

2.8.1.2 Impact on long-term viral suppression

HIV-1 drug resistance and genetic variability can undermine the ability to achieve and maintain long-term viral suppression, a key goal of HAART. The success of HAART depends on its ability to reduce the plasma HIV-1 RNA level to below detectable limits, typically defined as less than 50 copies/mL. Achieving undetectable viral load not only improves clinical outcomes but also reduces the risk of HIV transmission to others [4, 7, 36].

However, the emergence of drug-resistant strains can compromise the ability to maintain viral suppression. Once resistant variants emerge, they can continue replicating even in the presence of therapy, leading to a persistent viral load and increasing the risk of further resistance development. Over time, this can result in a cycle of drug resistance, treatment failure, and the need for more potent and complex regimens [4, 31].

Blips in viral load: Even in patients with good adherence to therapy, occasional transient increases in viral load, known as "viral blips," can occur. While blips are not always associated with the development of resistance, they can indicate low-level replication of drug-resistant variants within the viral quasi-species. Repeated or prolonged blips may signal an increased risk of virological failure and the need for closer monitoring [30, 33].

Durability of suppression: The durability of viral suppression is directly influenced by the virus's genetic variability and the patient's adherence to therapy. Patients who develop resistance may initially respond to second-line or third-line therapies, but the genetic diversity of the virus increases the likelihood that additional resistance mutations will emerge over time, leading to subsequent treatment failure [16, 20].

2.8.2 Limiting future treatment options

As HIV-1 develops resistance to antiretroviral drugs, the range of available treatment options becomes more limited. Drug-resistant variants can carry multiple mutations that confer resistance to entire classes of antiretroviral drugs, a phenomenon known as cross-resistance. Cross-resistance occurs when a single mutation or combination of mutations reduces the efficacy of several drugs within the same class or across different classes. For example, mutations in the reverse transcriptase gene can confer resistance to multiple nucleoside reverse transcriptase inhibitors (NRTIs), while mutations in the protease gene can lead to cross-resistance to protease inhibitors (PIs). The accumulation of resistance mutations limits the effectiveness of standard treatment regimens, requiring patients to switch to less commonly used drugs, which may have more side effects or be less accessible [12, 31, 35].

Second-line and third-line therapies: Patients who experience virological failure due to drug resistance often need to switch to second-line or third-line therapies. These regimens typically include drugs from different classes that have a higher genetic barrier to resistance, such as integrase strand transfer inhibitors (INSTIs) or boosted protease inhibitors (PIs). However, these regimens can be more expensive, have a higher pill burden, or require more frequent monitoring for side effects and drug interactions [23, 30, 34].

Impact of cross-resistance on treatment: Cross-resistance reduces the pool of effective drugs, making it more challenging to construct a viable regimen for patients with extensive drug resistance. In some cases, patients may develop resistance to all drugs within a specific class, necessitating the use of newer or experimental drugs. However, access to these drugs may be limited, especially in resource-constrained settings [19, 26, 29].

Transmitted drug resistance (TDR): Another concern is the transmission of drug-resistant HIV-1 strains to newly infected individuals. TDR occurs when a person acquires a strain of HIV-1 that already carries resistance mutations, often due to exposure to a partner with drug-resistant HIV. Individuals with TDR may have fewer treatment options from the outset, as their virus may already be resistant to one or more classes of antiretroviral drugs (**Figure 4**) [15, 20, 26].

2.8.3 Immune recovery and disease progression

The presence of drug-resistant HIV-1 can hinder immune recovery, increasing the risk of disease progression to acquired immunodeficiency syndrome (AIDS) and other HIV-related complications. HAART is designed to suppress viral replication, which allows the immune system, particularly CD4+ T cells, to recover. However, when drug-resistant variants emerge and viral suppression is not achieved, CD4+ T cell counts may fail to recover or may decline, leading to immunodeficiency [12, 22, 27].

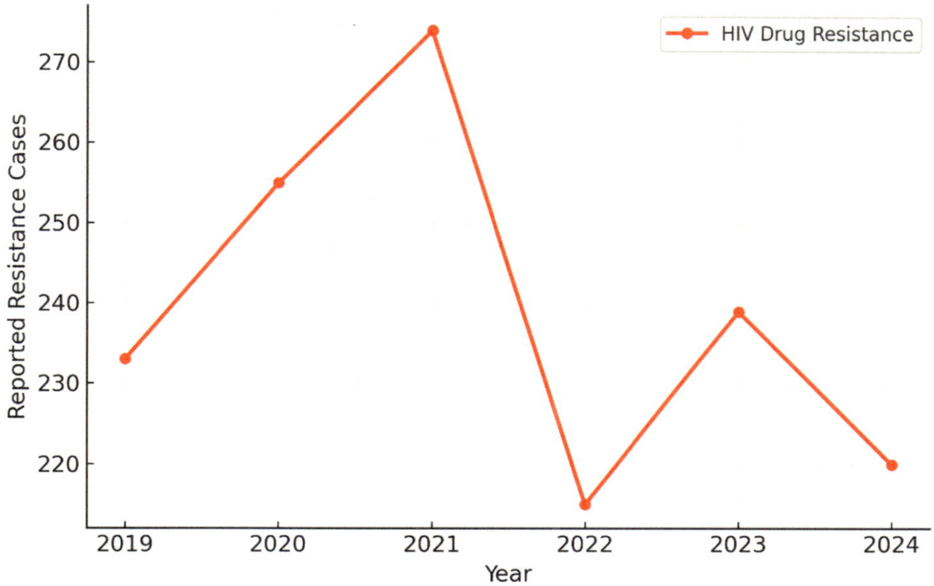

Figure 4.
Trends in HIV resistance research (2019–2024) (chart showing publication trends and key findings in HIV resistance studies).

Incomplete immune recovery: Even in patients who achieve partial viral suppression, the persistence of drug-resistant HIV-1 can limit the extent of immune recovery. The ongoing replication of resistant strains can prevent the full restoration of CD4+ T cell counts, leaving patients vulnerable to opportunistic infections and other complications of HIV-related immunosuppression [19, 36].

Increased risk of AIDS-related complications: Patients with drug-resistant HIV-1 who fail to achieve full viral suppression are at increased risk of developing AIDS-related complications, including opportunistic infections, malignancies, and neurocognitive disorders. The risk of disease progression is particularly high in patients with low CD4+ T cell counts or high viral loads despite therapy [12, 29, 36].

2.9 Future directions

As the global HIV epidemic continues, the evolution of drug-resistant strains and the virus's genetic variability pose ongoing challenges to effective long-term treatment. However, advances in antiretroviral therapy (ART) are constantly emerging to address these challenges. Future directions in HIV treatment focus on the development of next-generation antiretroviral drugs (ARVs), novel treatment strategies, and innovative approaches to overcoming resistance. Additionally, efforts to improve the accessibility and affordability of these therapies are critical, particularly in resource-limited settings where drug resistance is becoming more prevalent [16, 19, 25, 32].

2.9.1 Next-generation ARVs and resistance

The continuous development of next-generation antiretroviral drugs aims to improve the potency, tolerability, and convenience of HIV treatment while minimizing the risk of drug resistance. These drugs are designed to target HIV-1 in novel ways, offer higher genetic barriers to resistance, and provide alternative options for patients who have experienced treatment failure with existing therapies. Understanding the potential of these new drugs, along with their impact on drug resistance and clinical outcomes, is a key to shaping the future of HIV care [25, 32].

2.9.2 Characteristics of next-generation ARVs

Next-generation ARVs are being developed with several key characteristics in mind:

a. *Higher genetic barriers to resistance:* One of the most important goals in designing new ARVs is to create drugs with a higher genetic barrier to resistance, meaning that multiple mutations are required for the virus to develop resistance. Drugs with a high genetic barrier are less likely to result in treatment failure due to resistance, especially when used as part of combination therapy [16, 19].

b. *New mechanisms of action:* To combat resistance, next-generation ARVs often target different stages of the HIV replication cycle or inhibit viral proteins through novel mechanisms. By diversifying the ways in which the virus is attacked, these drugs can remain effective against strains that have developed resistance to older drugs [12, 17, 22].

c. *Improved pharmacokinetics and convenience*: Many next-generation ARVs are being designed for long-acting formulations that allow for less frequent dosing. Long-acting injectable ARVs, for example, can be administered monthly or even less frequently, improving patient adherence and reducing the likelihood of resistance emerging due to missed doses. Improved pharmacokinetics also ensure more consistent drug levels in the body, minimizing the risk of viral replication during periods of low drug concentration [31, 33, 35].

d. *Reduced side effects:* New ARVs aim to reduce the side effects commonly associated with the HIV treatment. By minimizing toxicity and adverse effects, next-generation drugs can improve patient adherence and reduce the risk of discontinuation, which in turn lowers the chances of resistance development [22, 30, 36].

2.9.3 New classes of ARVs

Several novel classes of ARVs are being developed or have recently entered the market, providing additional options for patients who have developed resistance to existing drugs. These new classes target different components of the HIV life cycle, offering fresh strategies for overcoming resistance [12, 34].

a. *Attachment inhibitors:* These drugs block HIV from attaching to the CD4 receptor on host cells, preventing the virus from entering the cell (**Table 3**). One example is fostemsavir, an attachment inhibitor approved for patients with multidrug-resistant HIV-1. By targeting the virus at the very first step of infection, attachment inhibitors offer a new mechanism to block viral replication in patients who have developed resistance to other ARV classes [12, 35].

b. *Maturation inhibitors:* Maturation inhibitors interfere with the final step of viral particle assembly, preventing the formation of mature, infectious virions.

Drug class	Mechanism of action	Advantage
Attachment inhibitors	Block viral entry	Effective against MDR HIV
Capsid inhibitors	Target capsid protein	Broad activity
bNAbs	Neutralize viral envelope	Long-acting potential

Table 3.
Characteristics of next-generation ARVs.

Although early drugs in this class, such as bevirimat, encountered challenges in the clinical development, ongoing research aims to refine maturation inhibitors to provide a potent option for patients with drug-resistant HIV [19, 26, 36].

c. *Capsid inhibitors:* Capsid inhibitors disrupt the viral capsid, a protein shell that encases the viral RNA and enzymes necessary for replication. Capsid inhibitors like lenacapavir offer a new approach by targeting the capsid at multiple stages of the viral life cycle. Lenacapavir, in particular, has shown promise as a long-acting drug that can be administered less frequently, making it an attractive option for improving adherence and reducing resistance (**Table 3**) [12, 20, 27].

d. *Broadly neutralizing antibodies (bNAbs)*: bNAbs are a novel therapeutic approach that harnesses the power of the immune system to neutralize a wide range of HIV-1 variants. Unlike traditional ARVs that target viral enzymes or proteins, bNAbs bind to conserved regions of the HIV envelope, preventing the virus from infecting host cells. Some bNAbs are being developed as part of combination therapy or as long-acting injectable treatments. By targeting conserved viral structures, bNAbs have the potential to reduce the emergence of drug-resistant strains and offer a new form of viral suppression (**Table 3**) [16, 30, 35].

2.9.4 Resistance to next-generation ARVs

Despite the promise of next-generation ARVs, resistance remains an ongoing concern. While newer drugs are designed to have higher genetic barriers to resistance, the evolution of the virus ensures that no drug is entirely immune to resistance development. Understanding the mechanisms by which HIV may develop resistance to next-generation drugs is crucial for optimizing their use in clinical practice [10, 11, 26].

a. *Resistance to attachment inhibitors:* Attachment inhibitors like fostemsavir have shown efficacy in patients with multidrug-resistant HIV-1. However, mutations in the HIV-1 envelope glycoprotein gp120 can potentially confer resistance to attachment inhibitors. These mutations may alter the structure of gp120, preventing the drug from effectively binding and blocking viral entry. To counter this, attachment inhibitors may need to be used in combination with other drugs to prevent the emergence of resistant variants [12, 23, 28].

b. *Resistance to capsid inhibitors:* Capsid inhibitors target the viral capsid protein, which plays a crucial role in several stages of the HIV life cycle. Resistance to capsid inhibitors may arise through mutations in the capsid protein that affect the drug's binding site. Early studies of lenacapavir have shown a low rate of resistance development, but ongoing monitoring is essential to identify any emerging patterns of resistance as the drug is used more widely in clinical settings [21, 27, 31, 33].

c. *Resistance to broadly neutralizing antibodies (bNAbs):* Although bNAbs target conserved regions of the HIV envelope, mutations in these regions can still arise, potentially allowing the virus to escape neutralization. However, the use of multiple bNAbs in combination, or pairing bNAbs with traditional ARVs, may help mitigate the risk of resistance. Researchers are also exploring ways to enhance the potency and breadth of bNAbs to ensure that they remain effective against diverse viral strains [12, 34, 36].

d. *Combination therapy and resistance:* One of the key strategies to prevent resistance with next-generation ARVs is the continued use of combination therapy. By combining drugs with different mechanisms of action, clinicians can reduce the likelihood that the virus will develop resistance to any one drug. For example, combining a capsid inhibitor with an integrase inhibitor and a reverse transcriptase inhibitor creates multiple barriers to viral replication, making it more difficult for resistance to emerge [12, 26, 36].

2.10 Long-acting formulations and resistance prevention

One of the most exciting developments in HIV treatment is the advent of long-acting ARVs, which can be administered monthly, quarterly, or even less frequently. Long-acting injectable formulations, such as the combination of cabotegravir and rilpivirine, offer a promising solution to the challenges of adherence, one of the primary drivers of resistance [12, 17, 23].

a. *Improving adherence:* Non-adherence to daily oral regimens are a major factor in the development of drug resistance. Long-acting formulations remove the burden of daily pill-taking, improving adherence and reducing the risk of missed doses. By maintaining consistent drug levels over extended periods, long-acting ARVs can suppress viral replication more effectively and lower the chances of resistance developing [12, 24, 31].

b. *Reducing viral replication windows:* Long-acting ARVs maintain therapeutic drug concentrations for longer periods, reducing the window of time during which the virus can replicate. This reduces the opportunity for resistant variants to emerge, particularly in patients who struggle with adherence to daily regimens. Additionally, long-acting drugs may simplify treatment for patients with resistance to multiple drug classes, offering a new option for achieving viral suppression [31, 34, 36].

3. Executive summary and conclusions

3.1 Executive summary

1. HAART has significantly improved HIV management, transforming it into a manageable chronic condition.

2. The high mutation rate of HIV-1 remains a primary challenge, driving drug resistance development.

3. Resistance mechanisms include both primary mutations and compensatory changes to maintain viral fitness.

4. Clinical implications of resistance include virological failure, reduced therapeutic options, and cross-resistance.

5. Advances in HAART focus on higher genetic barriers, long-acting formulations, and next-generation ARVs.

6. Monitoring and addressing adherence issues are critical for sustaining viral suppression.

7. Novel therapies, such as bNAbs and gene therapy, offer promising pathways for overcoming resistance.

8. Future strategies must integrate technology, expand access, and emphasize prevention and innovation.

4. Conclusions

The evolution of HIV-1 under HAART pressure is a dynamic and multifaceted process, shaped by the virus's genetic variability and its ability to develop drug resistance. This variability, driven by its rapid mutation rate and quasi-species population structure, enables HIV-1 to adapt to the selective pressures imposed by antiretroviral drugs, often leading to resistance. Drug resistance poses a significant challenge to the long-term success of antiretroviral therapy, potentially causing treatment failure and limiting future therapeutic options. Despite the potent viral suppression provided by HAART, issues such as adherence and access to treatment further complicate management. Understanding the mechanisms of resistance and genetic variability is critical for optimizing current treatment strategies and developing new therapies capable of outpacing viral evolution. Ongoing research into next-generation antiretrovirals, gene therapy, and cure strategies holds promise for overcoming the persistent challenges of HIV-1 drug resistance and ensuring the sustained effectiveness of treatment.

5. Future perspectives

1. Leveraging personalized medicine through advancements in sequencing technologies.

2. Developing cost-effective, long-acting therapies for widespread use.

3. Integrating global health strategies to ensure equitable access to treatments.

4. Expanding research into resistance mechanisms for newer ARVs.

5. Exploring synergistic therapies that combine traditional ARVs with immune-based approaches.

6. Enhancing resistance monitoring through AI-driven predictive tools.

7. Fostering global partnerships to tackle resistance emergence and spread.

Acknowledgements

Special thanks to our colleagues for their insightful feedback and to the organization for its unwavering support and resources throughout the research process. Without their collective contributions, this work would not have been possible. The authors also acknowledges the use of AI for language polishing of the manuscript.

Conflict of interest

No conflict of interest.

Author details

Bukhari ISah Shuaib[1*], Omosigho Omoruyi Pius[1] and Usman Aliyu Dutsinma[2]

1 Department of Medical Laboratory Science, Faculty of Applied Health Sciences, Edo State University Uzairue, Nigeria

2 Department of Microbiology, Faculty of Life Science, Bayero University, Kano, Nigeria

*Address all correspondence to: bukhari.shuaibu@edouniversity.edu.ng

References

[1] Odili VU, Obieche AO, Amibor KC. Adherence to antiretroviral therapy and its determinants among HIV-infected patients in Nigeria. Journal of Pharmacy Practice. 2017;**30**(3):291-295. DOI: 10.1177/0897190016633978

[2] Huynh K, Vaqar S, Gulick PG. HIV prevention. In: StatPearls [Internet]. Treasure Island (FL): StatPearls Publishing; 2024. Available from: https://www.ncbi.nlm.nih.gov/books/NBK470281/

[3] Bekker LG, Beyrer C, Mgodi N, Lewin SR, Delany-Moretlwe S, Taiwo B, et al. HIV infection. Nature Reviews. Disease Primers. 2023;**9**(1):42. DOI: 10.1038/s41572-023-00452-3. Erratum in: Nat Rev Dis Primers. 2023 Sep 11;9(1):48. doi: 10.1038/s41572-023-00464-z

[4] Matsuda K, Maeda K. HIV reservoirs and treatment strategies toward curing HIV infection. International Journal of Molecular Sciences. 2024;**25**(5):2621. DOI: 10.3390/ijms25052621

[5] Richman DD, Margolis DM, Delaney M, et al. The challenge of finding a cure for HIV infection. Science. 2009;**323**(5919):1304-1307

[6] Shin YH, Park CM, Yoon CH. An overview of human immunodeficiency Virus-1 antiretroviral drugs: General principles and current status. Infection & Chemotherapy. 2021;**53**(1):29-45. DOI: 10.3947/ic.2020.0100

[7] Wensing AM, Calvez V, Günthard HF, et al. 2017 update of the drug resistance mutations in HIV-1. Topics in Antiviral Medicine. 2017;**24**(4):132-133

[8] Wensing AM, Calvez V, Ceccherini-Silberstein F, et al. 2019 update of the drug resistance mutations in HIV-1. Topics in Antiviral Medicine. 2019;**27**(3):111-121

[9] Yeo JY, Goh G-R, Su CT-T, Gan SK-E. The determination of HIV-1 RT mutation rate, its possible allosteric effects, and its implications on drug resistance. Viruses. 2020;**12**(3):297. DOI: 10.3390/v12030297

[10] Shchemelev AN, Semenov AV, Ostankova YV, Naidenova EV, Zueva EB, Valutite DE, et al. Genetic diversity of the human immunodeficiency virus (HIV-1) in the Kaliningrad region. Problems of Virology. 2022;**67**(4):310-321. DOI: 10.36233/0507-4088-119

[11] Khan MA, Gupta KK, Singh SK. A review on pharmacokinetics properties of antiretroviral drugs to treat HIV-1 infections. Current Computer-aided Drug Design. 2021;**17**(7):850-864. DOI: 10.2174/1573409916666201006143007

[12] Apetroaei M-M, Velescu BȘ, Nedea MI, Dinu-Pîrvu CE, Drăgănescu D, Fâcă AI, et al. The phenomenon of antiretroviral drug resistance in the context of human immunodeficiency virus treatment: Dynamic and ever evolving subject matter. Biomedicine. 2024;**12**(4):915. DOI: 10.3390/biomedicines12040915

[13] International AIDS Society–USA Panel. Antiretroviral treatment of adult HIV infection: 2022 recommendations of the international AIDS society–USA panel. Journal of the American Medical Association. 2022;**304**(3):321-333. DOI: 10.1001/jama.2022.9784

[14] McLaren PJ, Fellay J. HIV-1 and human genetic variation. Nature

Reviews. Genetics. 2021;**22**:645-657. DOI: 10.1038/s41576-021-00378-0

[15] Barbehenn A, Shi L, Shao J, et al. Rapid biphasic decay of intact and defective HIV DNA reservoir during acute treated HIV disease. Nature Communications. 2024;**15**:9966. DOI: 10.1038/s41467-024-54116-1

[16] Martínez del Río J, Frutos-Beltrán E, Sebastián-Martín A, Lasala F, Yasukawa K, Delgado R, et al. HIV-1 reverse transcriptase error rates and transcriptional thresholds based on single-strand consensus sequencing of target RNA derived from *in vitro* transcription and HIV-infected cells. Journal of Molecular Biology. 2024;**436**(22):168815. DOI: 10.1016/j.jmb.2024.168815

[17] Ahmed RA, Adekoya KO, Onwuamah CK, Oboh BO, Iyer SS, Oluwatosin AS, et al. Mechanism of viral suppression among HIV elite controllers and long-term nonprogressors in Nigeria and South Africa. Viruses. 2022;**14**(6):1270. DOI: 10.3390/v14061270

[18] Sudderuddin H, Kinloch NN, Jin SW, et al. Longitudinal within-host evolution of HIV Nef-mediated CD4, HLA and SERINC5 downregulation activity: A case study. Retrovirology. 2020;**17**:3. DOI: 10.1186/s12977-019-0510-1

[19] Theys K, Libin P, Pineda-Peña AC, Nowé A, Vandamme AM, Abecasis AB. The impact of HIV-1 within-host evolution on transmission dynamics. Current Opinion in Virology. 2018;**28**:92-101. DOI: 10.1016/j.coviro.2017.12.001

[20] Hemelaar J, Elangovan R, Yun J, Dickson-Tetteh L, Fleminger I, Kirtley S, et al. Global and regional molecular epidemiology of HIV-1, 1990-2015: A systematic review, global survey, and trend analysis. The Lancet Infectious Diseases. 2019;**19**:143-155. DOI: 10.1016/S1473-3099(18)30647-9

[21] Godwe C, Goni OH, San JE, Sonela N, Tchakoute M, Nanfack A, et al. Phylogenetic evidence of extensive spatial mixing of diverse HIV-1 group M lineages within Cameroon but not between its neighbours. Virus Evolution. 2024;**10**(1):veae070. DOI: 10.1093/ve/veae070

[22] Banin AN, Tuen M, Bimela JS, Tongo M, Zappile P, Khodadadi-Jamayran A, et al. Development of a versatile, near full genome amplification and sequencing approach for a broad variety of HIV-1 group M variants. Viruses. 2019;**11**(4):317. DOI: 10.3390/v11040317

[23] Abongwa LE, Nyamache AK, Torimiro JN, et al. Human immunodeficiency virus type 1 (HIV-1) subtypes in the northwest region, Cameroon. Virology Journal. 2019;**16**:103. DOI: 10.1186/s12985-019-1209-6

[24] Vlasova-St. Louis I, Gorzalski A, Pandori M. Diagnostic applications for RNA-Seq technology and transcriptome analyses in human diseases caused by RNA viruses. In: Applications of RNA-Seq in Biology and Medicine. Rijeka: Intechopen; 2021. DOI: 10.5772/intechopen.99156

[25] Zhao J, Huang H, Lee S, Ragupathy V, Biswas S, Mbondji-wonje C, et al. Identification, genetic characterization and validation of highly diverse HIV-1 viruses for reference panel development. Viruses. 2021;**13**(7):1417. DOI: 10.3390/v13071417

[26] Ademuyiwa SEA, Saliu IO, Akinola BK, et al. Impact of highly active antiretroviral drug therapy (HAART) on biochemical, hematologic, atherogenic

and anthropometric profiles of human immunodeficiency virus patients at a tertiary hospital in Owo, Nigeria. Bulletin of the National Research Centre. 2022;**46**:263. DOI: 10.1186/s42269-022-00953-3

[27] Barbour JD, Hecht FM, Wrin T, et al. Higher CD4+ T cell counts associated with low viral pol replication capacity among treatment-naive adults in early HIV-1 infection. The Journal of Infectious Diseases. 2004;**190**(2):251-256

[28] Xu X, Luo L, Song C, et al. Survey of pretreatment HIV drug resistance and the genetic transmission networks among HIV-positive individuals in southwestern China, 2014-2020. BMC Infectious Diseases. 2021;**21**:1153. DOI: 10.1186/s12879-021-06847-5

[29] Sharma AL, Singh TR, Singh LS. Antiretroviral resistance, genotypic characterization and origin of human immunodeficiency virus among the infected wives of intravenous drug users in Manipur. Scientific Reports. 2018;**8**:15183. DOI: 10.1038/s41598-018-33636-z

[30] Heng X, Herrera AP, Song Z, et al. Retroviral PBS-segment sequence and structure: Orchestrating early and late replication events. Retrovirology. 2024;**21**:12. DOI: 10.1186/s12977-024-00646-x

[31] Günthard HF, Calvez V, Paredes R, Pillay D, Shafer RW, Wensing AM, et al. Human immunodeficiency virus drug resistance: 2018 recommendations of the International Antiviral Society–USA Panel. Clinical Infectious Diseases. 2019;**68**(2):177-187. DOI: 10.1093/cid/ciy463

[32] SeyedAlinaghi S, Afsahi AM, Moradi A, et al. Current ART, determinants for virologic failure and implications for HIV drug resistance: An umbrella review. AIDS Research and Therapy. 2023;**20**:74. DOI: 10.1186/s12981-023-00572-6

[33] Ge L, Luo Y, Li X, Hu Y, Sun L, Bu F, et al. Global, regional, and national prevalence of HIV-1 drug resistance in treatment-naive and treatment-experienced children and adolescents: A systematic review and meta-analysis. EClinicalMedicine. 2024;**10**:102859. DOI: 10.1016/j.eclinm.2024.102859

[34] Zhang Y, Wymant C, Laeyendecker O, Grabowski MK, Hall M, Hudelson S, et al. Evaluation of phylogenetic methods for inferring the direction of human immunodeficiency virus (HIV) transmission: HIV prevention trials network (HPTN) 052. Clinical Infectious Diseases. 2021;**72**(1):30-37. DOI: 10.1093/cid/ciz1247

[35] Temereanca A, Ruta S. Strategies to overcome HIV drug resistance-current and future perspectives. Frontiers in Microbiology. 2023;**14**:1133407. DOI: 10.3389/fmicb.2023.1133407

[36] Gandhi RT, Bedimo R, Hoy JF, et al. Antiretroviral drugs for treatment and prevention of HIV infection in adults: 2022 recommendations of the International Antiviral Society–USA panel. Journal of the American Medical Association. 2023;**329**(1):63-84. DOI: 10.1001/jama.2022.22246

Section 2

Optimizing HIV Care – Models, Interventions, and Co-Infections

Chapter 3

Recent Antiretroviral Therapy Models Implemented to Achieve Viral Suppression among People Living with Human Immunodeficiency Virus: A Systematic Review

Timothy Adejoh Attah, Solomon Jonathan Hussaini, Olamide Smart Aiyedogbon and Abubakar Adamu

Abstract

This is a systematic review of interventions adopted to improve viral outcomes of people living with human immunodeficiency virus (PLHIV). A search was performed on Science Direct and NCBI to select peer-reviewed articles based on the inclusion criteria. Titles, abstracts and full text were screened and relevant articles were selected into the review. Financial incentives were found to improve viral suppression among PLHIV. Psychosocial intervention demonstrated varying virologic outcomes. Differentiated service delivery including task shifting, community ART and home-based ART had higher viral suppression compared to standard care. Technology-related interventions including personalized text messaging, and computer-based counseling improve viral suppression. Other interventions like integrated HIV care services and monitoring of drug resistance improved or maintained viral suppression. Many interventions have been adopted and have improved virologic outcomes across the globe. However, Other research should be conducted to ensure more robust evidence for optimizing virologic outcomes of PLHIV.

Keywords: human immunodeficiency virus, antiretroviral therapy, universal ART coverage, viral suppression, HIV models

1. Introduction

Globally, antiretroviral therapy (ART) has been identified as the single significant cornerstone for maintaining the quality of life of people living with the human immunodeficiency virus (PLHIV). However, there are concerns about access to ART for PLHIV, especially in resource-limited areas. As of June 2021, the United Nations member State adopted the ambitious 95-95-95 target toward ensuring that 95% of PLHIV identify their status, 95% of PLHIV who know their status are on ART, and 95% of PLHIV on ART are virally suppressed by 2030 [1]. Globally, there are an estimated 40 million PLHIV, of which 95% know their status, 60% are on ART and 97% are virally suppressed [1, 2]. While there is significant progress in achieving these targets, there are disparities in coverage for ART among PLHIV, especially in low-and-middle-income countries (LMICs) where there are poor health infrastructures and resources to improve ART.

Given the need to address these limitations, there is a need for evidence-based interventions to improve access to ART for PLHIV. Numerous interventions and models have been adopted globally to first overcome the limitation of access to ART, ensure optimum health service delivery, and provide equitable and sustainable treatment for PLHIV while working toward achieving universal coverage in LMICs. However, it is important to understand the interventions that have been implemented to achieve a global decline in the prevalence of HIV. This will help to identify the successes and limitations of implemented strategies in addressing treatment gaps and achieving universal access to ART. Additionally, an adequate understanding of HIV interventions implemented can inform health policies to optimize treatment outcomes and achieve the ambitious UNAIDS targets.

Globally, the target toward eliminating HIV has focused on the prevention of new infections for those at risk and the improvement of the quality of life of PLHIV. Viral suppression, as indicated in the UNAIDS targets, is also critical in achieving the elimination of HIV across the globe by preventing transmission across the population and improving the quality of life among PLHIV. However, the major barrier to achieving viral suppression, especially in resource-limited areas, is the limited access to ART. Studies have shown that access to ART can be improved through various patient-centered and community-based models and interventions. However, some of these interventions have not been implemented in areas where they are needed or may help to improve access. According to the UNAIDS targets, about 23% of PLHIV do not have access to ART and 28% of ART are virally unsuppressed, despite 86% of PLHIV being aware of their status in 2023 [3]. This study reviews the non-pharmaceutic models and interventions implemented to achieve the third 95% of the UNAIDS targets since the global adoption of the 90-90-90 targets in 2014.

2. Method

2.1 Study design

A systematic review was conducted on NCBI and Science Direct to identify relevant articles on models adopted to achieve viral suppression among PLHIV across the globe.

2.2 Search term

Key search term used in this study were Effect of AND (((((((((((differentiated care) OR (community ART)) OR (antiretroviral therapy)) OR (community pharmacy)) OR (task shifting)) OR (multi-month dispensing)) OR (long acting injectables)) OR (universal test and treat)) OR (Same-Day ART Initiation)) OR (SMS reminder)) OR (mobile app)) OR (electronic pill boxes)) OR (Antiretroviral therapy to key populations)) AND (HIV treatment outcomes), Model of care for HIV.

2.3 Inclusion criteria

In this review, only studies conducted after the UNAIDS adoption of the 90-90-90 targets were included in this review. Thus, peer-reviewed randomized controlled trials (RCT) and quasi-experimental studies (QES) published between 2015 and 2024 that included drug delivery/access interventions to improve ART access and had information on viral suppression were selected for inclusion in the review. Studies conducted before 2015 that utilized non-experimental study designs or had no information on viral suppression of PLHIV were excluded from the review.

2.4 Search strategy

We conducted a literature search in four stages. First, titles were screened and selected for relevance and inclusion in the next stage. This was followed by the screening of abstracts in which studies relevant to the search were included for the final screening of full-text, while articles that were irrelevant or did not meet the inclusion criteria were excluded. Finally, the full text of selected abstracts was screened for relevance, and studies that met the inclusion criteria were finally selected for inclusion into the review.

2.5 Quality assessment

Quality assessment was performed on the full text of all studies included in this review based on the inclusion criteria. As a result, we adopted the JBI assessment checklist for RCT and QES and this assessment was conducted by one independent reviewer. The checklist for RCT assessed the quality of randomization in terms of selection, concealment of allocation, blinding of study participants, study implementers, and outcome evaluators, as well as the group similarities and quality of statistical analysis (**Table A1**) [4]. The quality assessment of QES included an assessment of the study objectives, inclusion of comparison groups, multiple measurements, and analysis of study outcomes (**Table A2**) [5].

2.6 Data extraction and synthesis

Data that were relevant to this review were extracted such as first authors, date of publication, country, number of participants, study design and study objectives, intervention administered, period of recruitment and follow-up, and number of participants in intervention and control group. Also, data on statistics of the viral outcomes of PLHIV were extracted and included in the review, and data was synthesized to answer the study objectives.

3. Result

Based on the search term, Science Direct produced 50,474 and NCBI 4784 outputs of which 208 titles from Science Direct, 750 from NCBI and 12 from references were selected for inclusion. A total of 18 duplicates were removed, resulting in 952 titles selected for inclusion. Abstracts of these titles were screened, of which 813 were excluded, and 139 abstracts were retrieved for full-text screening. 56 of the full text were excluded, and 83 were retrieved for the final screening. Of the 83 full-text articles selected, 36 had no information on viral suppression (VS) and were excluded from the review. Finally, 47 articles met the inclusion criteria and were selected for the review (**Figure 1**).

Of the 47 studies selected in this review, nine studies were conducted in the United States and seven in Zimbabwe. Six studies were conducted in South Africa and Tanzania and three in Kenya and Nigeria. Only two studies were conducted in Vietnam, Zambia and Uganda. Also, only one study was conducted in China, Malaysia, and Russia. Four studies were conducted on populations from different countries, of which two were conducted in Uganda and Kenya, one in South Africa and Zambia, and one in Ukraine, Vietnam and Indonesia) (**Table 1**).

Articles in this review assessed the effect of numerous non-pharmaceutical interventions on VS among PLHIV across the globe. These interventions were further divided into financial incentives, psychosocial support, differentiated care, the use of applications, and other interventions, respectively (**Figure 2**).

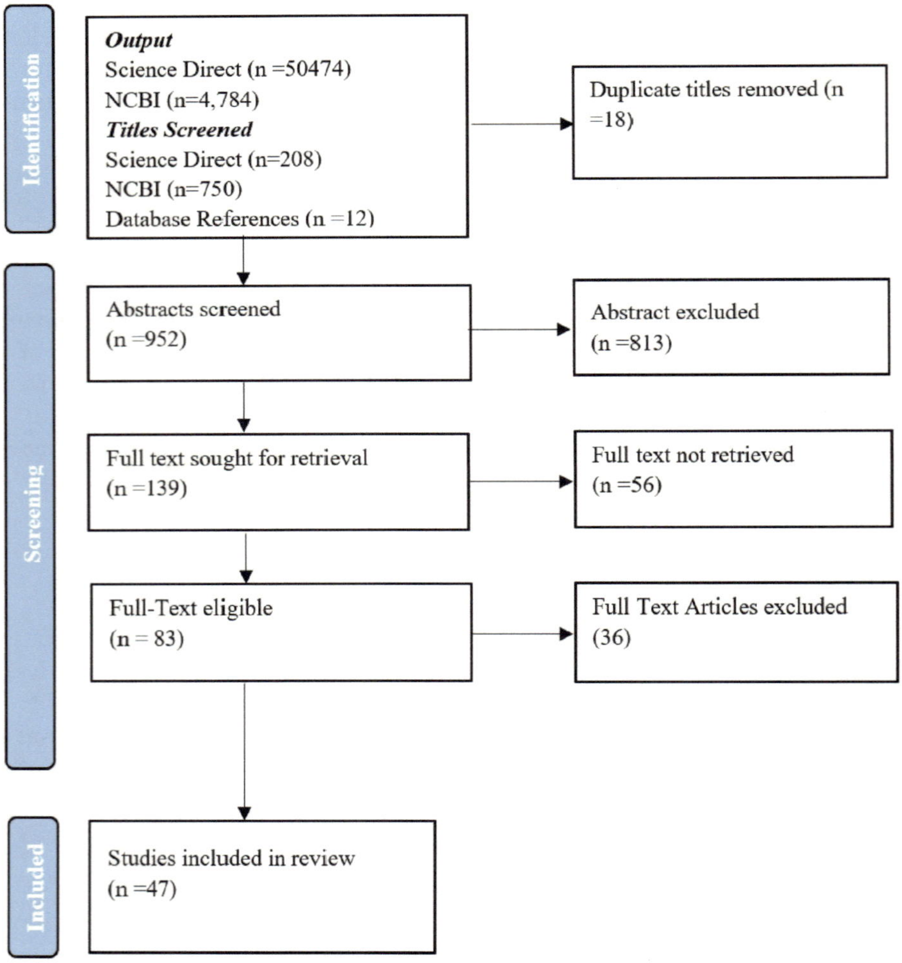

Figure 1.
PRISMA flowchart of articles selected for participation.

Country	Number of Studies
The United States	9
South Africa	6
Zambia	2
South Africa and Zambia	1
Nigeria	3
China	1
Uganda	2
Kenya	3
Uganda and Kenya	2
Tanzania	6
Zimbabwe	7
Vietnam	1
Malaysia	1
Russia	1
Ukraine, Vietnam and Indonesia	1
Zimbabwe and Lesotho	1

Table 1.
Number of articles selected by country of study.

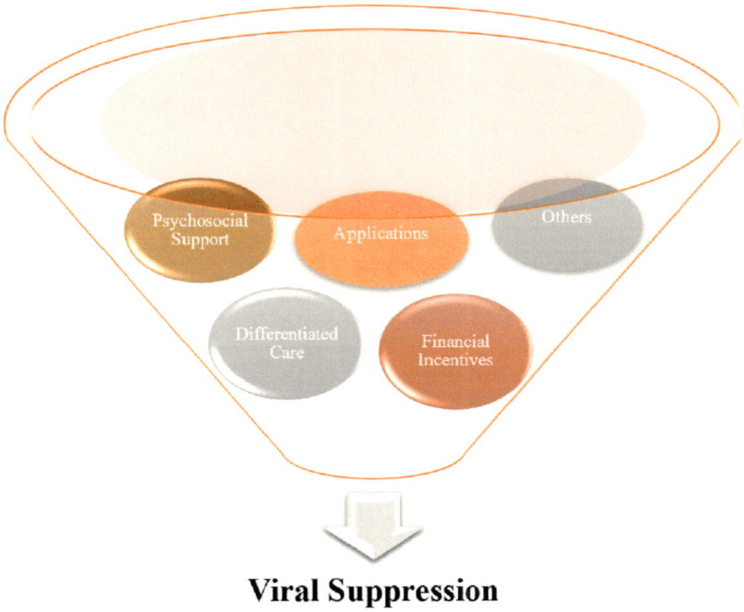

Figure 2.
Summary of interventions implemented to achieve viral suppression amongst PLHIV.

3.1 Financial incentives and viral suppression

A study conducted in Tanzania found that adults on ART who were administered short-term financial incentives had higher VS (84.9%) compared to those in standard care (80.6%) (RD: 4.6%, 95%CI: 1.5–11.0%) [6]. Also, another study in Tanzania found that after 6 months of intervention, small (93.8%) and large (94.9%) financial incentives increased the odds of VS when compared with standard care (87.1%) (aOR (small FI): 1.10, 95% CI: 1.03–1.17) [7]. In Nigeria, a study found that conditional economic incentives at 12 months increased VS from 21.8% at baseline to 31.9% after follow-up, while in the control group, VS reduced from 42.5% at baseline to 40.9% after follow-up (IRR: 1.01, 95% CI: 0.72–1.41), p:.96) [8]. Economic empowerment after 48 months was found to increase VS in a study conducted in Uganda (HR: 1.45, 995% CI: 1.07–1.95, p: .0155) [9] (**Table 2**).

3.2 Psychosocial support, training and viral suppression

In a study conducted in the United States, 58.4% of PLHIV on heart to heart intervention were virally suppressed compared to 40.0% of PLHIV on standard care, but this was not statistically significant (p > .05) [29]. Another study conducted in the US found that PLHIV on 6 months of Supporting Treatment Adherence Readiness through Training (START) intervention had higher VS (91.7%) compared to those on standard care (83.3%), but this finding was not statistically significant [27]. About 62% of the participants individuals motivated to Participate in Adherence, Care and Treatment (IMPACT) intervention were virally suppressed compared to 63% of those

Author, Date, Country, sample size	Study objective, and Study design	Model adopted, period of observation	Number per intervention group	HIV outcome
Limbada et al., 2022, South Africa and Zambia, 2489 [10]	A randomized controlled trial (RCT) to assess virological suppression of models of care compared to standard of care at 12 months after enrollment	Home-based delivery (HBD), adherence club (AC), Standard of care (SoC), 12 months	**Intervention** HBD: 852 (34%) AC: 856 (34%) **Control** SoC: 781(31%)	**12 months** **Known VS (Risk) (interv/SoC)** HBD: 61.3% AC: 57.0% SoC: 49.7% **20–24 months** **Estimated VS** HBD: 98.9% AC: 98.7% SoC: 99.2%
Fanfair et al., 2021, United States, 1893 [11]	An RCT to utilize Data to Care (D2C) model to identify out-of-care PLHIV and implement public health intervention to improve HIV care and outcome	Data to Care, August–October 2016(recruitment)-July 2018	**Intervention** D2C: 959 **Control** SoC: 935	**VS** D2C: 64.2% (*P:.22*) SoC: 61.5%
Samet et al., 2023, Russia, 225 [12]	An RCT to assess the effectiveness of multi-component pragmatic intervention, designed to link PWHIV in addiction treatment to HIV care and achieve viral load suppression	Linking Infectious and Narcology Care Part 2 (LINC-II) intervention, September 19 2018 to December 25, 2020	**Intervention** LINC-II: 111 **Control** SoC: 114	**12 months** **VS** LINC-II: 47% SoC: 23% Int/SoC aOR = 3.0, *P:.0039* RR = 2.1

Author, Date, Country, sample size	Study objective, and Study design	Model adopted, period of observation	Number per intervention group	HIV outcome
Patel et al., 2023, Kenya, 704 [13]	An RCT to evaluate if using higher frequency point of care (POC) viral load with targeted drug resistant monitoring (DRM) and clinical decision support (CDS) for children aged 1–14 years on ART could improve VS	POC viral load with targeted DRM testing and CDS (POCVL-DRM-CDS), March 2019–December 2020	**Intervention** POC-VL-DRM-CDS: 349 **Control** SoC: 355	**VS (< 1000 c/ml)** POCVL-DRM-CDS: 90.4% Control: 91.8% RR = 0.99, *P:.55*
Njau et al., 2024, Tanzania, 1990 [6]	A type 1 hybrid effectiveness-implementation cluster-randomized trial to evaluate the effectiveness of short-term financial incentives on viral suppression and retention in care among adults initiating ART at 32 HIV primary care clinics	Short-term financial incentives (S-TFI), May 28, 2021-March 7, 2022 (recruitment) to July 14, 2023 (intervention)	**Intervention** S-TFI: 1059 **Control** SoC: 931	**12 months VS (<1000 c/ml) and RiC** S-TFI: 84.9% SoC: 80.6% RD: 4.6% (1.5%–11.0%)
Fahey et al., 2020, Tanzania, 530 [7]	Three-arm parallel-group RCT to determine whether varied size of financial incentives for clinic attendance impact viral suppression among patients in ART.	Financial incentive for clinic attendance, April 24, 2018, to December 14, 2018 (randomization) to June 20, 2019 (follow-up)	**Intervention** 10,000TZS: 172 22,500 TZS: 174 **Control** No incentive: 184	**6 Months VS (<1000 c/ml)** 10,000TZS: 93.8% 22,500 TZS: 94.9% No incentive: 87.1% OR: 1.10/2500 TZS, (1.03–1.17) P = 0.0032
Wachira et al., 2023, Kenya, 328 [14]	A pilot RCT to assess the impact of a patient-centered intervention referred to as Enhanced Patient Care (EPC) on viral suppression among unsuppressed patients living with HIV in Kenya	Enhanced Patient-centered (EPC), provider-patient communication interventions, September 2017	**Intervention** PPC + EPC: 110 **Control** PPC+ SoC: 110 SoC: 108	**6 months VS** PPC + EPC: 84.4% (Ref) PPC+ SoC: 83.7% SoC: 64.4% aOR(PPC+ SoC) = 0.97 (0.45–2.08) aOR (SoC) = 0.36 (0.18–0.72)*
Drain et al., 2020, South Africa, 390 [15]	An open-label non-inferiority RCT to assess whether task shifting changed treatment and care outcomes for adults on ART when compared to standard care	Task Shifting (TS), February 24 to August 23, 2017 (recruitment)	**Intervention** TS: 195 **Control** SoC: 195	**12 months VS (<1000 c/ml)** TS: 90.0% SoC: 78.0% RD: 12.3% (5.1–19.5%) p-value:.0013
Ruel et al., 2023, Kenya and Uganda, 1549 [16]	A cluster-RCT to evaluate the effect of the SEARCH-Youth intervention in increasing the proportion of participants (15–24 years) with viral suppression	SEARCH-Youth intervention, January 2019 to March 1, 2022	**SEARCH-Youth:785 SoC: 764**	**24 months VS** SEARCH-Youth: 88% (85–92) SoC: 80% (77–84%) RR: 1.10 (1.03–1.16) p-value:.0019

Author, Date, Country, sample size	Study objective, and Study design	Model adopted, period of observation	Number per intervention group	HIV outcome
Mavhu et al., 2020, Zimbabwe, 500 [17]	A cluster-RCT to assess a peer-led differentiated service delivery intervention on HIV clinical and psychosocial outcomes among adolescents with HIV	Peer-led differentiated service delivery (PLDSD) intervention, August 15, 2016 to March 31, 2017 (recruitment) – 96 weeks	**Zvandiri: 212** **Control: 284**	**96 weeks** **VS ≥ 1000 c/μl** Zvandiri: 22% Control: 36% aPR: 058 (0.36–0.94) P-value:.03
Miller et al., 2018, Ukraine, Vietnam, Indonesia, 1004 [18]	A RCT to assess the feasibility of a future controlled trial based on incidence of HIV, enrollment, retentions, uptake of intervention and efficacy of an integrated and flexible intervention on ART use, viral suppression and medication-assisted treatment (MAT) use.	(HAPTEN 074) intervention comprising systems navigation, psychosocial counseling, and ART at any CD4 count. February 2015 to June 2016 (recruitment) – 12–24 months	**HTPN 074: 502** **SoC: 502**	**52 weeks** **VS (<40 c/ml)** HTPN: 74: 41% SoC: 24% PR: 1.7(1.3–2.2)
Ekwunife et al., 2022, Nigeria, 246 [8]	A cluster-RCT to evaluate the 1-year impact of conditional economic incentives and motivational interviewing on the health outcomes of adults living with HIV	Conditional economic incentives (CEI), December 1, 2018 to November 30, 2019	**CEI: 119** **Control: 127**	**12 Months** **VS (≤20 c/ml)** **CEI** Baseline: 21.8% After follow-up: 31.9% **Control** Baseline: 42.5% After follow-up: 40.9% IRR: 1.01 (0.72–1.41) p-value: .96
Kwaghe et al., 2023, Nigeria, 171 [19]	A facility-based retrospective study to evaluate the effectiveness of community-based private sector pharmacies to expand ART	Community pharmacy, June 2018 to May 2021	**Community pharmacy: 171**	**12 months** **Mean (median) VL** Pre: 399.3(20.0) Post: 259.5(20.0) t-test: −0.51 p-value: .612
Dakum et al., 2021, Nigeria, 251 [20]	A quasi-experimental study to assess the effect of community antiretroviral therapy (ART) group on immunologic, virologic and clinical outcomes of stable adult ART patients	Community ART group (CAG), August 2017 (recruitment) Follow-up: 1 year	**CAG: 251**	**12 months** **Log10 VL** Baseline: 3.5 (2.4–3.7) Follow-up: 3.7 (3.4–4.0) p-value:.40
Jiao et al., 2022, China, 576 [21]	An RCT to evaluate the effect of a differentiated digital intervention on ART adherence among men who have sex with men living with HIV	Differentiated digital intervention (DDI), October 19 2020–December 4 2020 (recruitment) Follow-up: October 19, 2020 to June 31, 2021	**DDI: 288** **SoC: 288**	**9 months** **VS** RR: 1.39 (0.64–3.05) *In-text message: 1.28 (0.15–10.59)* *Instant message: 0.85(0.27–2.62)* *Instant message + social media: 3.06(0.70–13.33)*

Author, Date, Country, sample size	Study objective, and Study design	Model adopted, period of observation	Number per intervention group	HIV outcome
Meya et al., 2022, Uganda, 1011 [22]	A quasi-experimental study to evaluate the impact of an intensive case management on HIV treatment outcomes	Intensive case management on HIV treatment outcomes, January 1, 2017 to December 31 2017 (pre-intervention), June 13, 2018 to June 30, 2019 (post-intervention)	**Pre-intervention: 606** **Post-intervention: 405**	**12 months** **VS** Pre-intervention: 87% Post-intervention: 87%
Fatti et al., 2020, Zimbabwe, 4800 [23]	A three-arm unblinded pragmatic non-inferiority trial to compare multi-month dispensing (MMD) with community ART refill groups (CARG) vs. SoC ART delivery	MMD, CARG, August 2017 to February 2018, 12 months (follow-up), 5	**Control arm (ART at three monthly intervals at facility): 1919** **Intervention arm 1 (ART at three monthly intervals in CARG with annual clinical visits and consolations): 1335** **Intervention arm 2 (ART at six-monthly intervals in CARG with annual clinic visits and consultations): 1546**	**12 months** **VS** 3MF: 99.1% 3MC: 99.7 6MC: 92.9% **RRR** 3MC: 1.0 (1.0–1.0) *p-value*:.49 6MC: 0.9 (0.9–1.0) *p-value*:.070
Cowan et al., 2018, Zimbabwe, 2883 [24]	A cluster-RCT to assess the efficacy of targeted combination intervention for female sex workers	Sisters Antiretroviral Prevention Programme—an Integrated Response (SAPPH-IRe), 2014–2016	**SAPPH-IRe: 1444** **SoC: 1439**	**24 months** **VS < 1000 c/ml** SAPPH-IRe: 72.0% (63.8–86.8%) SoC: 67.5% (61.4–73.1%) aRD: 5.3% (−4.0–14.6%) p-value:.20
Labhardt et al., 2018, South Africa, 278 [25]	Open-label 2-group RCT to determine whether offering same-day-based ART patients with HIV improves linkage to care and viral suppression in a rural high-prevalent setting	Same- day home-based ART (SDHBA), February 22, 2016 to September 17, 2017	**SDHBA: 138** **SoC: 140**	**VS < 100 c/ml** SDHBA: 50.4% SoC: 34.3% aD: 16.0% (4.4–27.2%) p-value:.007
Abdulrahman et al., 2017, Malaysia, 242 [26]	A single0-blind parallel-group RCT to determine the effectiveness of mobile phone reminders (SMS and telephone call reminders) and peer counseling in improving adherence and treatment outcomes among HIV-positive patients on ART	Mobile phone reminders and peer counseling (MPRPC), January 2014 to December 2014	**MPRPC: 121** **SoC: 121**	**12 months** **VL** *Baseline* MPRPC: 4.6 (4.44–4.78) SoC: 4.85 (4.67–5.02) *Follow-up* MPRPC: 1.4 (1.28–1.54) SoC: 1.76 (1.63–1.89) p-value:<.05

Author, Date, Country, sample size	Study objective, and Study design	Model adopted, period of observation	Number per intervention group	HIV outcome
Wagner et al., 2021, United States, 166 [27]	A multi-site RCT to examine the effect of supporting treatment adherence readiness through training (START) on ART adherence and virologic suppression	START, follow-up (24 months)	**START: 122** **SoC: 93**	**6 months** **VS (<200 c/ml)** START: 91.7% SoC: 83.3%% T: 1.17 p-value:.245 **24 months** **VS (<200 c/ml)** START: 67.3% SoC: 90.5% T: 1.12 p-value:.262
Fatti et al., 2021, Zimbabwe and Lesotho, 599 [28]	A cluster-RCT to determine effectiveness of community-based Differentiated Service Delivery (C-BDSD) for ART clients initiating DSD specifically within 12 months of ART initiation with single annual facility visits	C-BDSD, August 2017 to July 2019 (trial period)	**3MC (CAG for 3 months): 128** **6MC (CAG for 6 months): 259** **SoC: 212**	**VS** SoC: 99.3% 3MC: 98.6% 6MC: 98.1% 6MC: 98.1% RR (3MC/SoC): 0.99(0.97–1.02) p-value:.73 RR (6MC/SoC): 0.99 (0.96–1.01) p-value:.33 RR (6MC/SoC): 0.99 (0.96–1.03) p-value:.64
Gwadz et al., 2015, United States, 95 [29]	An RCT to examine a new culturally targeted multi-component intervention to address emotional, attitudinal, and social/ structural barriers to ART initiation and HIV car	Heart to Heart (HTH) intervention, 2012–2013	**HTH: 47** **SoC: 48**	**9 months** **VL** HTH: 58.4 SoC: 40.0 OR: 1.80 (0.55–6.08) p-value:.296
Ssewamala et al., 2019, Uganda, 288 [9]	A cluster-RCT to test the effect of household economic empowerment (EE) among adolescents living with HIV in affected communities	EE, 2012–2018, 48 months (follow-up)	**EE: 158** **SoC: 130**	**48 months** **VS** Hazard ratio: 1.45 (1.07–1.95) p-value:.0155
Mageda et al., 2023, Tanzania, 45 [30]	A preliminary cluster-RCT to evaluate the effectiveness of a community-based interventions (Konga model) in addressing factors contributing to low viral load suppression among children living with HIV	Konga (patient-centered interventions aimed at reducing the viral loads of children in terms of measurements, follow-up 6 months)	**Konga: 15** **SoC: 30**	**VL** Konga: 165.13 Control: 516.70 F: 4.3 p-value:.0414

Author, Date, Country, sample size	Study objective, and Study design	Model adopted, period of observation	Number per intervention group	HIV outcome
Hickey et al., 2020, Uganda and Kenya, 6190 [31]	A community cluster-RCT to evaluate the effect of streamlines care among those who newly linked to care after universal HIV testing in the SEARCH trial among adolescents and adults (age > 15 years) PLHIV	SEARCH (differentiated service delivery model), addresses structural barriers to care, improve relationships between patients and clinic and enhance patient and clinician knowledge of HIV and ART, 2013–2017	**SEARCH: 3394** **SoC: 2796**	**36 years** **VS (<500 c/ml** SEARCH: 67% SoC: 47% RR: 1.41 (1.05–1.91)
Schnall et al. 2022, United States, 200 [32]	A randomized controlled efficacy trial to determine the efficacy of WiseApp, a user-centered design mHealth intervention to improve ART adherence and suppression in PLWH	WiseApp (self-management app for PLWH), January 31, 2018, to April 13, 2021 (recruitment), 6 months (follow-up)	**WiseApp: 99** **SoC: 101**	**6 months** **VS WiseApp/SoC** p-value:.89
Fox et al., 2019, South Africa, 569 [33]	A cluster-RCT to evaluate five differentiated ART delivery interventions and present an evaluation of two strategies (adherence club and decentralized medication delivery) for clinically stable patients	Adherence club and decentralized medication delivery, enrollment: March 2017 to March-2017, 18 months (follow-up)	**AC: 275** **SoC: 294** **DMD: 232** **SoC: 346**	**18 months** **VS (<250 c/ml)** **Adherence Club** AC: 95.2% SoC: 94.4% RD: 0.4% (−6.2–7.0%) **Decentralized ART delivery** DMD: 98.4% SoC: 90.2% RD: 2.9% (−4.2–10.0%)
Hayes et al., 2019, Zambia, 48,301 [34]	A community RCT to report results from the HPTN 071 (PopART) and its impact on viral suppression	HTPN 071 (PopART), 2013–2018	**Arm A: 12671** **Arm B: 1304** **Arm C (SoC): 12399**	**VS** Arm A: 71.9% Arm B: 67.5% Arm C: 60.2% **Adjusted VS prevalence** Arm A: 1.16 (0.99–1.47) p-value:.071 Arm B: 1.08 (0.92–1.27) p-value:.297

Author, Date, Country, sample size	**Study objective, and Study design**	**Model adopted, period of observation**	**Number per intervention group**	**HIV outcome**
Go et al., 2020, Vietnam, 440 [35]	A 3-group RCT to determine the effect of two clinic-based behavioral interventions of varying intensity on alcohol use and viral suppression among individuals with HIV and hazardous alcohol use	Combines intervention (Personalized feedback, Consideration of pros and cons, Strategies for managing risky moods and situations for alcohol use, Alcohol refusal skills, Managing negative thoughts), brief intervention (personalized feedback, consideration of pros and cons, Strategies for managing risky moods and situations for alcohol use). Recruitment (March 2016 to May 2017), follow-up (12 months)	**Combined: 147** **Brief: 147** **SoC: 146**	**VS < 20 c/ml** Combined: 83.1% Brief: 80.2% SoC: 78.1% p-value:.06
Wohl et al., 2017, United States, 405 [36]	An RCT to compare the effects of impact multi-dimensional intervention to promote care engagement after release, to standard care on sustaining viral suppression after community re-entry	individuals motivated to Participate in Adherence, Care and Treatment (impact), March 2012 to February 2015 (recruitment), 24 weeks (follow-up)	**impact: 195** **SoC: 186**	**VS < 50 c/ml** impact: 62% SoC: 63% aOR: 0.92 (0.55–1.54)
DiPrete et al., 2019, United States, 405 [37]	An impact trial aims to examine differences in ART adherence between study arms and provide an overall assessment of adherence to ART after release from prison	impact, recruitment (March 2012 to February 2015), follow-up (24 weeks)	**impact: 195 (128)** **SoC: 186 (125)**	**6 months VS** impact: 61% SoC: 61% p-value: >.05
Brijkumar et al., 2020, South Africa, 109 [38]	A quasi-experimental study to determine if viral load monitoring could be improved and the impact on these changes on virologic suppression	Package intervention (fact sheet on demographics, serial CD4 count and VL results; clinical chart in flow sheet for monthly visit; viral load sample log, and high viral load register), May 2014 to July 2018	**Mkuze: 37** **Jozini: 60** **Bethesda: 12** **109**	**VS (effect)** **Mkuze** Total effect: 39.3% p-value:<.001 RR: 0.89 p-value:<.01 **Bethesda CDC** Total effect: 9.3% p-value:.12 RR: 0.86 p-value:.58 **Jozini** Total effect: 36.2% p-value:<.01 RR: 1.70 p-value:<.01

Author, Date, Country, sample size	Study objective, and Study design	Model adopted, period of observation	Number per intervention group	HIV outcome
Sunpath et al., 2022, South Africa, 116 [39]	A pre and post implementation evaluation to assess the impact of the viral load champion model adapted to identify support and coordinate the management of individuals with virologic failure on first-line ART in a setting with limited electronic-abased record capacity	Viral load champion model, initiation (January 2017), pre-intervention (December 2015 to December 2016), post-intervention (January 2017 to December 2017)	**Post-intervention: 56** **Pre-intervention: 60**	**12 months** **VF** **Median** Post-intervention: 19,443 (4751–82,910) Pre-intervention: 16,963 (5621–144,977) p-value:.64
Abuogi et al., 2022, Kenya. 1331 [40]	A cluster-RCT to evaluate the impact of two evidence-based behavioral interventions on adherence and retention in women living with HIV	Mother-Infant Visit Adherence and Treatment Engagement (MOTIVATE), December 2015 to August 2017	**Text messaging only: 263** **Community mentor mothers: 262** **SoC: 253** **cMM and text message: 264**	**12 months** **VS** **Text messaging only** Undetectable: 44.9% <1000 c/ml: 6.6% >1000c/ml: 5.7% **Community mentor mothers** Undetectable: 44.8% <1000 c/ml: 9.4% >1000c/ml: 4.8% **cMM and text message** Undetectable: 51.5% <1000 c/ml: 7.8% >1000c/ml: 4.5% **SoC** Undetectable: 44.4% <1000 c/ml: 16.5% >1000c/ml: 6.0% **P-value:.900**
Cowan et al., 2024, Zimbabwe, 2137 [41]	A cluster open label-RCT to evaluate the effect of risk-differentiated, peer-led support for female sex workers	May 15, 2019, to June 1, 2019 (enrollment), follow-up (June 1, 2019, to December 13, 2021)	**AMETHIST: 2131** **SoC: 2137**	**12 months** **VS** Intervention: 93.5% SoC: 88.8% aRD: 5·8% (2·7 to 8·8)
Ferrand et al., 2017, Zimbabwe, 470 [42]	An open-label RCT to assess the effect of community-based support for caregivers of HIV-infected children and adolescents who are key mediators to children engaging with care, on treatment outcomes	Community-based support (CBS), January 2013 to January 2015 (enrollment), follow-up (12 months)	**CBS: 166** **SoC: 168**	**12 months** **VF (≥400 c/mL) or mortality** CBS: 33% SoC: 49% aOR: 0.46 (0.23–0.89) p-value:.02
Garofalo et al., 2016, United States, 133 [43]	An open-label RCT of a two-way personalized daily text messaging intervention to improve adherence to ART among 105 poorly adherent HIV-positive adolescents and young adults (16–29 years)	Personalized daily text message reminders (PDTMR), October 2010 to February 2014	**PDTMR: 51** **SoC: 54**	**6 months** **VS ≤ 75 copies/ml** PDMTR: 70.8% SoC: 60.0% p-value:.272

Author, Date, Country, sample size	**Study objective, and Study design**	**Model adopted, period of observation**	**Number per intervention group**	**HIV outcome**
Dow et al., 2020, Tanzania, 128 [44]	A random group treatment trial to establish the feasibility and acceptability of the *Sauti ya Vijana (SYV): the voice of youth,* intervention in preparation for a fully powered effectiveness trial	*Sauti ya Vijana (SYV): the voice of youth,* June 2016 to July 2017, 6 months (follow-up)	SYV: 55 SoC: 38	**6 months** **VS < 400 c/ml** SYV Baseline: 65.8% F6 months: 65.8% SoC Baseline: 64.8% 6 months: 74.5%
Pascoe et al., 2019, South Africa, 730 [45]	A cluster-RCT to evaluate the effect of a package of adherence interventions on the impact of fast-track treatment initiation counseling (FTIC) on ART initiation, adherence and retention	fast-track treatment initiation counseling (FTIC), January to December 2016 (recruitment), 18 months (follow-up)	FTIC: 362 SoC: 368	**18 months** **VS < 400 c/ml** FTIC Pre-intervention: 61.1% Pos intervention: 61.0% SoC Pre-intervention: 61.2% Post-intervention: 63.9% RD:-0.1 (−1.9–1.8%) DID: −1.9% (−9.1–5.4%)
Wagner et al., 2023, Tanzania, 391 [46]	A cluster-RCT to assess whether integrated depression care model is superior to usual care in helping women adhere to each step of the PMTCT care continuum, via depression alleviation	Maternal depression treatment in HIV (M-DEPTH), 42 months (follow-up)	M-DEPTH: 191 SoC: 200	**VS < 400 c/ml** OR: 1.19 (0.73–1.93)
Mukama et al., 2024, Uganda, 2668 [47]	An RCT to evaluate the effectiveness and responsiveness of differentiated HIV/AIDS service delivery models (DSDMs) implemented to enhance ART access and outcomes for patients while addressing Tuberculosis (TB)-HIV integration	Facility-based individual management (FBIM) model and non-facility base individual management (nFBIM) such as; CCLAD, CDDP, and the FTDR models. 12 months	**Intervention** CCLAD: 689(26.3%) CDDP: 546(20.9%) FTDR: 735(28.1%) **Control** FBIM: 645(24.7%)	**12 months** **VS** CCLAD: 94.4% CDDP: 96.9% FTDR: 96.5% FBIM: 76.3%
Melvin and Gipson. 2019, United States, 231 [48]	A quasi-experimental study to determine whether an integrated model of HIV care influenced linkage to health care, adherence to antiretroviral therapy, and viral load	Integrated HIV care services(ICS) model, January 1, 2015 through December 31, 2017	**ICS: 231**	**VS** 2015: 59% 2016: 76% 2017: 81%
Haas et al., 2023, Zimbabwe, 516 [49]	An RCT to assess the effect of a lay health worker-led psychological intervention on ART adherence, virologic suppression, and mental health symptoms.	Friendship Bench (FB) intervention, October 2018 to December 2019.	**Intervention** FB: 244 **Control** SC: 272	**VS, Odd Ratio** Month 6: 2.20(0.79 to 6.14) Month 12: 1.60(0.42 to 6.05)

Author, Date, Country, sample size	Study objective, and Study design	Model adopted, period of observation	Number per intervention group	HIV outcome
Chinoda et al., 2020, Zimbabwe, 840 [50]	An RCT to evaluate the feasibility and effectiveness of a peer-led mental health support intervention on virological suppression, mental health and quality of life in ALHIV.	CATS-PST Model, 48 weeks	**CATS**: 840	**12 months** **VF at Baseline** CATS-PST: 840(30%) CATS Standard: 840(43%) Power: 85% at 0.25 coefficient variation **VF post-intervention** CATS-PST: 840(8%) CATS Standard: 840(16%) Power: 87%
Kurth et al., 2016, USA, 494 [51]	RCT aimed to adapt a computer-based counseling tool, demonstrated to reduce HIV-1 viral load and sexual risk transmission in a population of English-speaking adults, for use during routine clinical visits for an HIV-positive Spanish-speaking population (CARE+ Spanish)	Computer Assessment and Rx Education for HIV-positives (CARE+), 12 months	**Intervention** CARE+ Spanish: 226 **Control** SC: 207	**Detectable VL** CARE+ Spanish: 78 (34.5) Control: 76 (36.7) P = .69
Lyatuu et al., 2022, Tanzania, 3341 [52]	An RCT to evaluate the effect of a peer-mother interactive program on PMTCT outcomes among pregnant women on antiretroviral treatment (ART) in routine healthcare	peer-mother adherence support, January 1, 2018, to December 31, 2019	**Intervention** Peer-mother: 1957 **Control** SoC: 1384	**VS (95%CI)** Peer-mother: 92% (91, 93) SoC: 91% (90, 92)

Note: VS = viral suppression; SoC = standard of care; p = significance level at 95% confidence; + = plus; RD = risk difference; RR = risk ratio; aRR = adjusted risk ratio; DID = difference in difference; aOR = adjusted odds ratio; <=less than; c/ml = copies per miles; VF = viral failure; VL = viral load; ul = micro liters.

Table 2.
Viral load outcomes in studies selected into the review.

on standard care aOR: 0.92 (0.55–1.54) [36]. Another study in the US found that after 24 weeks of incarceration, VS among those on IMPACT intervention (61%) was not significantly different from participants on standard care (61%) (p-value>.05) [37]. Also, friendship bench intervention increased the odds of VS at six months (aOR: 2.2, 95%CI: 0.79–6.14) and at 12 months (aOR: 1.6, 95% CI: 0.42–6.05) when compared to baseline VS [49]. Peer-led mental health support intervention reduced the proportion of adolescents that were virally suppressed from 30% at baseline to 8% after 48 weeks and also for standard care from 43–16%) [50]. An intervention titled Voice of Youth was found to maintain the proportion of youths with VS at baseline and 6 months after implementation (65.8%) compared to 64.8%/74.5% in the standard group [44]. Maternal depression treatment in HIV (M-DEPTH) was also found to increase the odds of VS in the intervention group compared to the control (OR: 1.19, 95%CI: 0.73–193) in a study conducted on women on prevention of mother-to-child transmission care [46].

In Vietnam, the combined intervention of personalized feedback, consideration of pros and cons, and strategies for managing risky moods and situations for alcohol increased VS (83.1%) compared to brief intervention (80.2%) and standard care (78.1%), but this was not statistically significant (p:.06). A study was conducted in Ukraine, Vietnam and Indonesia found that the HTPN medication-assisted treatment increased VS (74.41%) compared to standard care (24%) (PR: 1.7, 95%CI: 1.3–2.2) [18]. A study conducted in Uganda and Kenya also found that adolescents and adult PLHIV in the SEARCH program had a higher proportion of participants with VS (47%) compared to those in standard care (47%) after three years of follow-up (RR: 1,41, 95% CI: 1.05–1.91) [26, 31]. Another study conducted in Kenya and Uganda found that PLHIV aged 15–24 years on SEARCH-Youth intervention (life stage assessment tool, alternative clinic access, rapid viral load feedback and provider E-collaborative) had higher proportion of participants that were virally suppressed (88%, 95% CI: 85–92%) compared to standard care (80%, 95% CI: 77–84%) (RR: 1.10, 95% CI: 1.03–1.16, p:.0019). Fast-track treatment initiation counseling maintained VS at about 61% of the PLHIV while standard care increased from 61.2% to 63.9% after 18 months [45]. Another study found that 72.0% (63.8–86.8%) of the female sex workers on sisters antiretroviral prevention program were virally suppressed compared to 5.3% (−4.0–14.6%) on standard care after 12 months of follow-up (aRD: 5.3%, 95%CI: −4.0-14.6%, p:.20) (**Table 2**) [24].

3.3 Differentiated care and viral suppression

A study conducted in South Africa reported that 90% of PLHIV on task shifting intervention had VS compared to those on standard care (78%) (RD: 12.3%, 95% CI: 5.1–19.5%, p:.0013) [15]. Another study found a higher proportion of PLHIV on same-day, home-based ART (SDHBA) (50.4%) was virally suppressed compared to standard care (34.3%) (aRD: 16.0%, 95%CI: 4.4–27.2%, p:.007) [25]. Adherence club (95.2%) produced higher PLHIV with VS compared to standard care (94.4%) (RD: 0.4, 95%CI: −6.2-7.0%), and decentralized ART delivery (98.4%) produced more virally suppressed PLHIV compared to standard care (90.2%) for clinically stable PLHIV (RD: 2.9, 95%CI: −4.2-10.0%) [33]. A total of seven studies were conducted in Zimbabwe, of which one study found that after 96 weeks, a lesser proportion of adolescents PLHIV on peer-led differentiated service delivery (22%) had VS compared to those on standard care (36%) (aPR: 0.58, 95%CI: 0.36–0.94, p:.03) [17]. Another RCT on multi-month dispensing with community ART refill groups found that those on three monthly intervals (99.7%) and six-monthly intervals (92.9%) community ART had higher VS compared to those in standard care (99.1%) [3MC (RR): 1.0(1.0–1.0), p:.49; 6MC: 92.9%(0.9–1.0), p:.70] [23]. Another similar study found that female sex workers on differentiated peer-led support intervention had higher VS (93.5%) compared to standard care (aRD: 5.8% (2.7–8.8) after 12 months of follow-up [41]. Community-based support for caregivers of HIV-infected children and adolescents reduced the proportion of participants with VS (33%) compared to those on standard care (49%) with statistical significance (aOR: 0.46, 95%CI: 0.23–0.89, p:.02) [42]. A study found that there was a slightly higher proportion of pregnant women on ART in the peer-mother adherence group with VS (92%, 95%CI: 91–93%) compared to those on standard care (91%, 95%CI: 90–92%) [52]. Community pharmacy in a study conducted in Nigeria was also found to reduce the viral load from 399.3c/ml in pre-intervention to 259.5c/ml in pos intervention, but this was not significant (p:.612) [19]. According to a study in Nigeria, although there was an increase in the $\log_{10}$ of the viral load of stable PLHIV on ART after one year of intervention (log_{10}: 3.5/3.7, p:.40), this was not statistically significant [20]. A study conducted in South Africa and Zambia found that a higher proportion of the participants in home-based delivery (61.3%) and adherence club (57.0%) had VS compared to those on standard care (49.7%) ART [10]. However, this study also found that although >95% of participants in home-based delivery (98.9%) and adherence club (98.7%) had VS, this was lower compared to those in standard of care (99.2%) [10]. Another study in Zimbabwe and South Africa found that three months (98.6%) and six months (98.1%) community ART delivery compared to standard care (99.3) did not significantly affect VS after 12 months of follow-up [RR(3MC): 0.99, 95%CI: 0.97–1.02, p:.73; RR(6MC): 0.99, 95%CI: 0.96–1.03, p:.64)] [28]. A community-based intervention targeted to reduce viral load in children (Konga) in Tanzania also found that after 6 months of intervention, the viral load was significantly lower in the intervention group (165.13 c/ml) compared to standard care (516.70 c/ml) (F: 4.3, p:.0414) (**Table 2**) [30].

3.4 Application, daily reminder and viral suppression

A study found that there was no significant difference in the VS of PLHIV in the United States on WiseApp self-management app intervention compared to the standard ART care (p:.89) [32]. Personalized daily text message reminder (PDTMR) in the United States had an insignificantly higher proportion of PLHIV with VS compared to those on standard care (70.8%/60.0%, p:.272) [43]. Another study found that the proportion of PLHIV with detectable viral load in the computer-based counseling tool group compared to standard care was insignificant (34.5%/36.7%, p:.69) [51]. A quasi-experimental study conducted to identify support and coordinate management of individuals with virologic failure on first-line ART in electronic-based limited settings found a significantly lower risk of VS in PLHIV on package intervention (fact sheet on demographics, serial CD4 count and viral load result, clinical chart in flowsheet for monthly visit, viral load sample log and high viral load register) in Mkuze (RR: 0.89, $p < .01$) and a higher risk in Jozini (RR: 1.70, $p < .01$) compared to standard care [38]. However, this variation in VS was insignificant in Bethesda CDC (RR: 0.86, p:.58) [38]. A study found that mother-infant visit adherence and treatment engagement through text messaging only (44.9%), community mentor mothers (44.8%) and joint intervention (51.5%) resulted in higher proportion of women on ART with undetectable viral load compared to those on standard care (44.4%) although insignificant [40]. A study found that after enhanced patient-centered, provider-patient communication intervention for six months, participants in the intervention group receiving standard care (83.7%) were less likely to be virally suppressed than those receiving provider-patient communication and enhanced patient care (84.4%), although insignificant [14]. However, those in only standard care (64.4%) were less likely than those receiving provider-patient communication and enhanced patient care to be virally suppressed (aOR: 0.36, 95%CI: 0.18–0.72) [14]. In China, differentiated digital intervention was found to increase the risk of VS when compared with those on standard care for in-text messages (RR: 1.28, 95%CI: 0.15–10.59) and instant message+social media (RR: 3.06, 95%CI: 0.70–13.33) while instant message only (RR: 0.85, 95%CI: 0.27–2.62) reduced the risk of VS [21]. In Malaysia, a study found that mobile phone reminders significantly reduced viral load from 4.6 (4.44–4.78) at baseline to 1.4 (1.28–1.54) after follow-up compared to 4.85 (4.67–5.02) at baseline and 1.76 (1.63–1.89) after follow-up for those on standard care ($p < .05$) [16]. A study conducted in the United States found that there was no significant difference in VS of participants who were enrolled in data-to-care intervention (64.5%) compared to those on standard ART care (61.5%) (*P = 0.22*) (**Table 2**) [11].

3.5 Other interventions and viral suppression

A quasi-experimental study conducted in the United States also found an increase in the proportion of PLHIV on integrated HIV care services intervention with VS (81%) in 2017 compared to 76% in 2016 and 59% in 2015 [48]. In Kenya, a study found that after one year of follow-up, a similar proportion of PLHIV in Point of Care viral load with targeted drug resistance monitoring and clinical decision support (90.4%) compared to standard care (91.8%) were virally suppressed (RR = 0.99, P:.55) [13]. In a study conducted in Uganda, the rate of VS was maintained after 1 year post-intensive case management on HIV treatment intervention at 87% [22]. A study conducted in Russia found that 12 months VS was higher in PLHIV integrated into linking infectious disease and narcology intervention (47%) compared to those on standard care (23%) (aOR: 3.0, p:.0039) (**Table 2**) [12].

4. Discussion

This study reviewed the impact of the implementation of HIV-service delivery interventions since the adoption of the 90–90-90 targets in 2014 with a focus on viral suppression. However, these targets were further reviewed to the global achievement of 95–95-95 targets, with the third target indicating that 95% of PLHIV on ART are virally suppressed. In recent times, innovative approaches have been implemented to improve service delivery for PLHIV with a focus on ease of access, efficiency and quality in improving patient outcomes.

HIV-service delivery models such as the DSD have recently been adopted across resource-limited regions as a patient-centered approach that provides targeted strategies to eliminate the barriers of access to care such as finance, convenience and distance from healthcare facilities. This review found that the implementation of various differentiated care service delivery was effective in improving virologic outcomes of PLHIV [53, 54]. The model is a patient-centered approach that provides a peer support system that fosters community engagement and mitigates the impact of stigma associated with assessing HIV care in healthcare facilities. As a result, DSD promotes retention in care and adherence to treatment. A meta-analysis of studies conducted in over 26 countries across the globe found that PLHIV with optimal adherence had a lower risk of virologic failure compared to their counterparts with sub-optimal adherence [55]. Another study conducted in South Africa reported a relationship between optimal adherence to treatment and virologic suppression among PLHIV [56]. The implementation of differentiated service delivery for PLHIV could potentially promote personalized care while maintaining optimal clinical outcomes and achieving the UNAIDS target of eliminating HIV.

Financial incentives have been identified as one of the interventions implemented to promote access to care for numerous diseases including HIV. This intervention is efficient in resource-limited areas where the transportation cost can negatively affect the ability to access healthcare and health-seeking behaviors among PLHIV. All studies in our review found that financial incentives or economic empowerment was effective in improving VS among PLHIV [7, 57, 58]. This intervention eliminates the economic barrier to accessing healthcare services and the dependence on personal funds to access ART, while promoting adherence to treatment. Findings from studies in this review is consistent with other studies that have found financial incentives to be effective in improving uptake of ART, adherence and retention in care [59, 60].

In our review, numerous psychosocial interventions were implemented for PLHIV on ART. These interventions have been implemented to provide psychosocial support that promotes health-seeking behaviors among PLHIV, especially high-risk populations like incarcerated inmates, adolescents and pregnant women. Although these interventions have been shown to improve VS, it is important that context-specific psychosocial interventions are implemented to meet the needs of the PLHIV at risk of virologic failure and address psychological barriers to adherence and retention in care.

Technology has been found to improve the ART cascade as studies have shown improvement in the effectiveness of ART among PLHIV. However, some technological interventions did not significantly improve VS among ART clients. Technology can help track the level of adherence to medication and clinical outcomes of PLHIV, and data can be used to implement strategies to promote health outcomes among non-adherent clients or those with poor HIV outcomes. However, the feasibility of this strategy in some regions remains a major concern as there are limited resources to effectively implement this intervention.

Studies included in this review found promising potentials of the various models in improving VS among PLHIV. However, there are some unmet needs impeding the achievement of the third 95 of the UNAIDS target. Some of the key challenges include the inability to scale-up these service delivery interventions across all high-risk populations due to limited resources in LMIC. Additionally, stigma remains a major concern that continuously prevent PLHIV from seeking care especially among high-risk populations like transgender, men sleeping with men and sex workers. Adolescent HIV care is faced with challenges like the poor institution of adolescent-friendly clinics and adherence support, which prevent care seeking for this group and poor adherence to treatment. Also, there are limited studies on HIV care and the risk of chronic co-morbidities among aging population. The occurrence of disease pandemics has been found to disrupt HIV care delivery. Thus, the decentralized model could play a significant role in eliminating this barrier. It is important that these gaps are addressed with much focus on implementing a patient-centered approach that promotes trust, equity, quality, innovation and a strengthened health system.

Some limitations were identified in this review. This study is a review and, as a result does not infer causality. Also, various cut-offs were adopted to determine viral suppression, which prevented comparison between groups and across similar interventions. The study was conducted on various sub-populations and during different follow-up periods, limiting our ability to compare between groups. However, this review is robust and provides information on the models adopted to improve VS across the globe. This data can be used in implementing public health strategies aimed at improving virological outcomes of PLHIV while achieving the third 95 of the UNAIDS ambitious targets.

5. Conclusion

This review finds that supportive interventions tailored toward the needs of PLHIV such as financial incentives and differentiated service delivery, can enhance VS among PLHIV. While psychosocial support and technology-driven interventions improved VS of PLHIV, there is no significant evidence for these findings; hence, there is a need for further research to better understand these approaches. Thus, it is recommended that health programs improve financial incentives, especially in resource-limited settings, to improve access to ART. Also, strategies should be implemented to promote the decentralization of ART into communities, as this can help improve clinical outcomes and barriers to accessing care. It is important that comprehensive psychosocial support systems and initiatives to empower PLHIV are developed and implemented to strengthen adherence to ART and improve virologic outcomes. Additionally, there is a need to set adequate structures that promote good health outcomes among aging populations, and it is important that adolescent-friendly clinics and social support interventions are implemented to promote trust in the health system and improve HIV care-seeking behaviors among adolescent populations.

Acknowledgements

The authors acknowledge the independent reviewer for assessing the quality of studies included in this review.

Conflict of interest

The authors declare no conflict of interest.

Appendix

	[10]	[11]	[12]	[13]	[6]	[7]	[14]	[15]	[16]	[17]	[18]	[8]	[21]	[23]	[24]	[25]	[26]	[27]	[28]	[29]	[9]
1. Was true randomization used for assignment of participants to treatment groups?	👍	👍	👍	👍	👍	👍	👍	👍	👍	👍	👍	👎	👍	👍	👍	👍	👍	👍	👍	👍	👍
2. Was allocation to treatment groups concealed?	👎	👍	👎	👎	👎	👍	👎	👍	👎	👍	👎	👍	👍	👎	👎	👍	👍	👎	👎	👎	👎
3. Were treatment groups similar at the baseline?	👍	👍	👍	👍	👍	👍	👍	👍	👍	👍	👍	👎	👍	👍	👍	👍	👍	👍	👍	👍	👍
4. Were participants blind to treatment assignment?	👎	👎	👎	👎	👎	👎	👎	👍	👎	…	👎	👍	👎	👎	👎	👎	👎	👎	👎	👎	👎
5. Were those delivering treatment blind to treatment assignment?	👎	👍	👎	👎	👎	👎	👎	👍	👎	👎	👎	👍	👍	👎	👎	👎	👍	👎	👎	👎	👎
6. Were outcomes assessors blind to treatment assignment?	👎	…	👎	👍	👎	👎	👎	👍	👍	👍	👎	👎	👍	👎	👍	👎	👍	👎	👎	👎	👎
7. Were treatment groups treated identically other than the intervention of interest?	👍	👍	👍	👍	👍	👍	👍	👍	👍	👍	👍	👍	👍	👍	👍	👍	👍	👍	👍	👍	👍
8. Was follow-up complete and if not, were differences between groups in terms of their follow-up adequately described and analyzed?	👍	👍	👍	👍	👍	👍	👍	👍	👍	👍	👍	👍	👍	👍	👍	👍	👍	👍	👍	👍	👍
9. Were participants analyzed in the groups to which they were randomized?	👍	👍	👍	👍	👍	👍	👍	👍	👍	👍	👍	👍	👍	👍	👍	👍	👍	👍	👍	👍	👍

	[10]	[11]	[12]	[13]	[6]	[7]	[14]	[15]	[16]	[17]	[18]	[8]	[21]	[23]	[24]	[25]	[26]	[27]	[28]	[29]	[9]
10. Were outcomes measured in the same way for treatment groups?	👍	👍	👍	👍	👍	👍	👍	👍	👍	👍	👍	👍	👍	👍	👍	👍	👍	👍	👍	👍	👍
11. Were outcomes measured in a reliable way?	👍	👍	👍	👍	👍	👍	👍	👍	👍	👍	👍	👍	👍	👍	👍	👍	👍	👍	👍	👍	👍
12. Was appropriate statistical analysis used?	👍	👍	👍	👍	👍	👍	👍	👍	👍	👍	👍	👍	👍	👍	👍	👍	👍	👍	👍	👍	👍
13. Was the trial design appropriate, and any deviations from the standard RCT design (individual randomization, parallel groups) accounted for in the conduct and analysis of the trial?	👍	👍	👍	👍	👍	👍	👍	👍	👍	👍	👍	👍	👍	👍	👍	👍	👍	👍	👍	👍	👍

	[30]	[31]	[32]	[33]	[34]	[35]	[36]	[37]	[40]	[41]	[42]	[43]	[44]	[45]	[46]	[47]	[61]	[49]	[50]	[51]	[52]
1. Was true randomization used for assignment of participants to treatment groups?	👍	👍	👍	👍	👍	👍	👍	👍	👍	👍	👍	👍	👍	👍	👍	👍	👍	👍	👍	👍	👍
2. Was allocation to treatment groups concealed?	👍	👎	👍	👎	👎	👎	👎	👎	👍	👍	👍	👍	👍	👎	👎	👎	👍	👎	👎	👎	👎
3. Were treatment groups similar at the baseline?	👍	👍	👍	👍	👍	👍	👍	👍	👎	👍	👍	👍	👍	👍	👍	👍	👍	👍	👍	👍	👍
4. Were participants blind to treatment assignment?	👎	👎	👍	👎	👎	👎	👎	👎	👎	👎	👎	👎	👎	👎	👎	👍	👎	👎	👍	👍	👎
5. Were those delivering treatment blind to treatment assignment?	👎	👎	👎	👎	👎	👍	👎	👎	👎	👎	👎	👎	👍	👎	👎	👎	👎	👍	👍	👎	👎

	[10]	[11]	[12]	[13]	[6]	[7]	[14]	[15]	[16]	[17]	[18]	[8]	[21]	[23]	[24]	[25]	[26]	[27]	[28]	[29]	[9]
6. Were outcomes assessors blind to treatment assignment?	👎	👍	👎	👎	👎	👍	👎	👎	👎	👍	👍	👎	👍	👎	👎	👎	👎	👍	👍	👎	👎
7. Were treatment groups treated identically other than the intervention of interest?	👍	👍	👍	👍	👍	👍	👍	👍	👍	👍	👍	👍	👍	👍	👍	👍	👍	👍	👍	👍	👍
8. Was follow-up complete and if not, were differences between groups in terms of their follow-up adequately described and analyzed?	👍	👍	👍	👍	👍	👍	👍	👍	👍	👍	👍	👍	👍	👍	👎	👍	👍	👍	👍	👍	👍
9. Were participants analyzed in the groups to which they were randomized?	👍	👍	👍	👍	👍	👍	👍	👍	👍	👍	👍	👍	👍	👍	👍	👍	👍	👍	👍	👍	👍
10. Were outcomes measured in the same way for treatment groups?	👍	👍	👍	👍	👍	👍	👍	👍	👍	👍	👍	👍	👍	👍	👍	👍	👍	👍	👍	👍	👍
11. Were outcomes measured in a reliable way?	👍	👍	👍	👍	👍	👍	👍	👍	👍	👍	👍	👍	👍	👍	👍	👍	👍	👍	👍	👍	👍
12. Was appropriate statistical analysis used?	👍	👍	👎	👍	👍	👍	👍	👍	👍	👍	👍	👍	👍	👍	👍	👍	👍	👍	👍	👍	👍
13. Was the trial design appropriate, and any deviations from the standard RCT design (individual randomization, parallel groups) accounted for in the conduct and analysis of the trial?	👍	👍	👍	👍	👍	👍	👍	👍	👍	👍	👍	👍	👍	👍	👍	👍	👍	👍	👍	👍	👍

Table A1.
Quality assessment of randomized controlled trials.

	[19]	[20]	[62]	[22]	[38]	[39]	[48]	[63]
1. Is it clear in the study what is the 'cause' and what is the 'effect' (i.e. there is no confusion about which variable comes first)?	👍	👍	👍	👍	👍	👍	👍	👍
2. Were the participants included in any comparisons similar?	👎	👎	👎	👎	👎	👍	👎	👍
3. Were the participants included in any comparisons receiving similar treatment/care, other than the exposure or intervention of interest?	👎	👎	👎	👎	👎	👍	👎	👍
4. Was there a control group?	👎	👎	👎	👎	👎	👎	👎	👎
5. Were there multiple measurements of the outcome both pre and post the intervention/exposure?	👎	👎	👍	👎	👎	👍	👎	👎
6. Was follow-up complete and if not, were differences between groups in terms of their follow-up adequately described and analyzed?	👍	👍	👍	👍	👍	👍	👍	👍
7. Were the outcomes of participants included in any comparisons measured in the same way?	👍	👍	👍	👍	👍	👍	👍	👍
8. Were outcomes measured in a reliable way?	👍	👍	👍	👍	👍	👍	👍	👍
9. Was appropriate statistical analysis used?	👍	👍	👍	👍	👍	👍	👍	👍

Table A2.
Quality assessment of quasi-experimental studies.

Author details

Timothy Adejoh Attah[1]*, Solomon Jonathan Hussaini[1], Olamide Smart Aiyedogbon[2] and Abubakar Adamu[1]

1 Department of Physical and Life Sciences, National Space Research and Development Agency, FCT-Abuja, Nigeria

2 AIDS Prevention Initiative, Public Health Initiatives, FCT-Abuja, Nigeria

*Address all correspondence to: attah_adejoh@yahoo.com

References

[1] UNAIDS. Understanding measures of progress towards the 95-95-95 HIV testing, treatment and viral suppression targets [Internet]. 2023. Available from: https://www.unaids.org/sites/default/files/media _asset/progress-towards-95-95-95_en.pdf

[2] UNAIDS, WHO. HIV. 2024. Available from: https://www.who.int/data/gho/data/themes/hiv-aids#:~:text=Globally%2C%2039.9%20 million%20%5B36.1%E2%80% 93,considerably%20between%20 countries%20and%20regions

[3] HIV.gov. The global impact of HIV and AIDS. Available from: https://www.hiv.gov/hiv-basics/overview/data-and-trends/global-statistics#:~:text=UNAIDS%20 reports%20that%20in%202023,72%20 %25%20were%20virally%20suppressed

[4] JBI. Checklist for randomized controlled trials critical appraisal tools for use in JBI systematic reviews [Internet]. 2020. Available from: https://jbi.global/sites/default/files/2020-08/Checklist_for_RCTs.pdf

[5] JBI. Checklist for quasi-experimental studies (non-randomized experimental studies) critical appraisal tools for use in JBI systematic reviews [Internet]. 2020. Available from: https://jbi.global/sites/default/files/2020 -08/Checklist_for_Quasi-Experimental_Appraisal_Tool.pdf

[6] Njau PF, Katabaro E, Winters S, et al. Impact of financial incentives on viral suppression among adults initiating HIV treatment in Tanzania: A hybrid effectiveness–implementation trial. The Lancet HIV. 2024;**11**:e586-e597

[7] Fahey CA, Njau PF, Katabaro E, et al. Financial incentives to promote retention in care and viral suppression in adults with HIV initiating antiretroviral therapy in Tanzania: A three-arm randomised controlled trial. The Lancet HIV. 2020;**7**:e762-e771

[8] Ekwunife OI, Anetoh MU, Kalu SO, Ele PU, Egbewale BE, Eleje GU. Impact of conditional economic incentives and motivational interviewing on health outcomes of adolescents living with HIV in Anambra state, Nigeria: A cluster-randomised trial. Contemporary Clinical Trials Communications. 2022;**30**:100997

[9] Ssewamala FM, Dvalishvili D, Mellins CA, et al. The long-term effects of a family based economic empowerment intervention (Suubi+adherence) on suppression of HIV viral loads among adolescents living with HIV in southern Uganda: Findings from 5-year cluster randomized trial. PLoS One. 2020;**15**:e0228370

[10] Limbada M, Macleod D, Situmbeko V, et al. Rates of viral suppression in a cohort of people with stable HIV from two community models of ART delivery versus facility-based HIV care in Lusaka, Zambia: A cluster-randomised, non-inferiority trial nested in the HPTN 071 (PopART) trial. Lancet HIV. 2022;**9**:e13-e23

[11] Fanfair RN, Khalil G, Williams T, et al. The cooperative Re-engagement controlled trial (CoRECT): A randomised trial to assess a collaborative data to care model to improve HIV care continuum outcomes. The Lancet Regional Health - Americas. 2021;**3**:100057

[12] Samet JH, Blokhina E, Cheng DM, et al. Rapid access to antiretroviral therapy, receipt of naltrexone, and

strengths-based case management versus standard of care for HIV viral load suppression in people with HIV who inject drugs in Russia (LINC-II): An open-label, randomised controlled trial. Lancet HIV. 2023;**10**:e578-e587

[13] Patel A. Antiretroviral therapy in resource-limited settings: Challenges and opportunities. Journal of Antivirals & Antiretrovirals. 2024;**16**:336

[14] Wachira J, Genberg B, Mwangi A, Chemutai D, Braitstein P, Galarraga O, et al. Wilson I (2022) impact of an enhanced patient care (EPC) intervention on viral suppression among patients living with HIV in Kenya. Journal of Acquired Immune Deficiency Syndromes. 1999;**90**:434

[15] Drain PK, Dorward J, Violette LR, et al. Point-of-care HIV viral load testing combined with task shifting to improve treatment outcomes (STREAM): Findings from an open-label, non-inferiority, randomised controlled trial. The Lancet HIV. 2020;**7**:e229-e237

[16] Ruel T, Mwangwa F, Balzer LB, et al. A multilevel health system intervention for virological suppression in adolescents and young adults living with HIV in rural Kenya and Uganda (SEARCH-youth): A cluster randomised trial. The Lancet HIV. 2023;**10**:e518-e527

[17] Mavhu W, Willis N, Mufuka J, et al. Effect of a differentiated service delivery model on virological failure in adolescents with HIV in Zimbabwe (Zvandiri): A cluster-randomised controlled trial. The Lancet Global Health. 2020;**8**:e264-e275

[18] Miller WC, Hoffman IF, Hanscom BS, et al. A scalable, integrated intervention to engage people who inject drugs in HIV care and medication-assisted treatment (HPTN 074): A randomised, controlled phase 3 feasibility and efficacy study. The Lancet. 2018;**392**:747-759

[19] Kwaghe A, Kwaghe V, Habib Z, Kwaghe G, Ilesanmi O, Ekele B, et al. Stigmatization and psychological impact of COVID-19 pandemic on frontline healthcare Workers in Nigeria: A qualitative study. BMC Psychiatry. 2021;**21**:518

[20] Dakum P, Ajav-Nyior J, Attah TA, et al. Effect of community antiretroviral therapy on treatment outcomes among stable antiretroviral therapy patients in Nigeria: A quasi experimental study. PLoS One. 2021;**16**:e0250345

[21] Jiao K, Wang C, Liao M, Ma J, Kang D, Tang W, et al. A differentiated digital intervention to improve antiretroviral therapy adherence among men who have sex with men living with HIV in China: A randomized controlled trial. BMC Medicine. 2022;**20**:341

[22] Meya DB, Kiragga AN, Nalintya E, et al. Impact of an intensive facility-community case management intervention on 6-month HIV outcomes among select key and priority populations in Uganda. AIDS Research and Therapy. 2022;**19**:62

[23] Fatti G, Ngorima-Mabhena N, Mothibi E, et al. Outcomes of three-versus six-monthly dispensing of antiretroviral treatment (ART) for stable HIV patients in community ART refill groups: A cluster-randomized trial in Zimbabwe. Journal of Acquired Immune Deficiency Syndromes. 2020;**84**:162-172

[24] Cowan FM, Davey C, Fearon E, et al. Targeted combination prevention to support female sex workers in Zimbabwe accessing and adhering to antiretrovirals for treatment and prevention of HIV

(SAPPH-IRe): A cluster-randomised trial. The Lancet HIV. 2018;**5**:e417-e426

[25] Labhardt ND, Ringera I, Lejone TI, Klimkait T, Muhairwe J, Amstutz A, et al. Effect of offering same-day ART vs usual health facility referral during home-based HIV testing on linkage to care and viral suppression among adults with HIV in Lesotho: The CASCADE randomized clinical trial. JAMA. 2018;**319**:1103

[26] Abdulrahman SA, Rampal L, Ibrahim F, Radhakrishnan AP, Kadir Shahar H, Othman N. Mobile phone reminders and peer counseling improve adherence and treatment outcomes of patients on ART in Malaysia: A randomized clinical trial. PLoS One. 2017;**12**:e0177698

[27] Wagner GJ, Hoffman R, Linnemayr S, Schneider S, Ramirez D, Gordon K, et al. START (supporting treatment adherence readiness through training) improves both HIV antiretroviral adherence and viral reduction, and is cost effective: Results of a multi-site randomized controlled trial. AIDS and Behavior. 2021;**25**:3159-3171

[28] Fatti G, Ngorima-Mabhena N, Tiam A, Tukei BB, Kasu T, Muzenda T, et al. Community-based differentiated service delivery models incorporating multi-month dispensing of antiretroviral treatment for newly stable people living with HIV receiving single annual clinical visits: A pooled analysis of two cluster-randomized trials in southern Africa. Journal of the International AIDS Society. 2021;**24**(Suppl 6):e25819

[29] Gwadz M, Cleland CM, Applegate E, et al. Behavioral intervention improves treatment outcomes among HIV-infected individuals who have delayed, declined, or discontinued antiretroviral therapy: A randomized controlled trial of a novel intervention. AIDS and Behavior. 2015;**19**:1801-1817

[30] Mageda K, Kulemba K, Kilimba E, Katalambula LK, Kapologwe N, Petrucka P. Effectiveness of a community-based intervention (Konga model) to address factors contributing to low viral load suppression among children living with HIV in Tanzania: A preliminary, cluster, randomized clinical trial report. BMC Public Health. 2023;**23**:1280

[31] Hickey MD, Ayieko J, Kwarisiima D, et al. Improved viral suppression with streamlined care in the SEARCH study. Journal of Acquired Immune Deficiency Syndromes. 2020;**85**:571-578

[32] Schnall R, Sanabria G, Jia H, Cho H, Bushover B, Reynolds NR, et al. Efficacy of an mHealth self-management intervention for persons living with HIV: The WiseApp randomized clinical trial. Journal of the American Medical Informatics Association. 2023;**30**:418-426

[33] Fox MP, Pascoe S, Huber AN, Murphy J, Phokojoe M, Gorgens M, et al. Adherence clubs and decentralized medication delivery to support patient retention and sustained viral suppression in care: Results from a cluster-randomized evaluation of differentiated ART delivery models in South Africa. PLoS Medicine. 2019;**16**:e1002874

[34] Hayes RJ, Donnell D, Floyd S, et al. Effect of universal testing and treatment on HIV incidence - HPTN 071 (PopART). The New England Journal of Medicine. 2019;**381**:207-218

[35] Go VF, Hutton HE, Ha TV, et al. Effect of 2 integrated interventions on alcohol abstinence and viral suppression among Vietnamese adults with hazardous alcohol use and HIV: A randomized clinical trial. JAMA Network Open. 2020;**3**:e2017115

[36] Wohl DA, Golin CE, Knight K, et al. A randomized controlled trial of an intervention to maintain suppression of

HIV viremia following prison release: The imPACT trial - JAIDS Ms. No.: QAIV16986. Journal of Acquired Immune Deficiency Syndromes (1999). 2017;**75**:81

[37] DiPrete BL, Pence BW, Golin CE, Knight K, Flynn PM, Carda-Auten J, et al. Antiretroviral adherence following prison release in a randomized trial of the imPACT intervention to maintain suppression of HIV viremia. AIDS and Behavior. Sep 2019;**23**(9):2386-2395

[38] Brijkumar J, Johnson BA, Zhao Y, et al. A packaged intervention to improve viral load monitoring within a deeply rural health district of South Africa. BMC Infectious Diseases. 2020;**20**:836

[39] Sunpath H, Pillay S, Hatlen T, Murphy RA, Marconi VC, Moosa M-YS, et al. A nurse-led intervention to improve management of virological failure in public sector HIV clinics in Durban, South Africa: A pre- and post-implementation evaluation. South African Medical Journal. 2021;**111**:299-303

[40] Abuogi LL, Onono M, Odeny TA, et al. Effects of behavioural interventions on postpartum retention and adherence among women with HIV on lifelong ART: The results of a cluster randomized trial in Kenya (the MOTIVATE trial). Journal of the International AIDS Society. 2022;**25**:e25852

[41] Cowan FM, Machingura F, Ali MS, et al. A risk-differentiated, community-led intervention to strengthen uptake and engagement with HIV prevention and care cascades among female sex workers in Zimbabwe (AMETHIST): A cluster randomised trial. The Lancet Global Health. 2024;**12**:e1424-e1435

[42] Ferrand RA, Simms V, Dauya E, et al. The effect of community-based support for caregivers on the risk of virological failure in children and adolescents with HIV in Harare, Zimbabwe (ZENITH): An open-label, randomised controlled trial. Lancet Child Adolescent Health. 2017;**1**:175-183

[43] Garofalo R, Kuhns LM, Hotton A, Johnson A, Muldoon A, Rice D. A randomized controlled trial of personalized text message reminders to promote medication adherence among HIV-positive adolescents and young adults. AIDS and Behavior. 2016;**20**:1049-1059

[44] Dow DE, Mmbaga BT, Gallis JA, Turner EL, Gandhi M, Cunningham CK, et al. A group-based mental health intervention for young people living with HIV in Tanzania: Results of a pilot individually randomized group treatment trial. BMC Public Health. 2020;**20**:1358

[45] Pascoe SJ, Fox MP, Huber AN, Murphy J, Phokojoe M, Gorgens M, et al. Differentiated HIV care in South Africa: The effect of fast-track treatment initiation counselling on ART initiation and viral suppression as partial results of an impact evaluation on the impact of a package of services to improve HIV treatment adherence. Journal of the International AIDS Society. 2019;**22**:e25409

[46] Wagner GJ, Gwokyalya V, Faherty L, et al. Effects of M-DEPTH model of depression care on maternal HIV viral suppression and adherence to the PMTCT care continuum among HIV-infected pregnant women in Uganda: Results from a cluster randomized controlled trial at pregnancy completion. AIDS and Behavior. 2023;**27**:2902-2914

[47] Mukama SC, Nakawesi JS, Bindeeba DS, Ezajobo S, Mugisa A, Senyimba C, et al. Evaluating antiretroviral therapy service delivery models through lot quality assurance sampling in Central Uganda. HIV AIDS (Auckl). 2024;**16**:337-354

[48] Melvin SC, Gipson J. The open arms healthcare Center's integrated HIV care services model. Preventing Chronic Disease. 2019;**16**:E135

[49] Haas AD, Kunzekwenyika C, Manzero J, et al. Effect of the friendship bench intervention on antiretroviral therapy outcomes and mental health symptoms in rural Zimbabwe: A cluster randomized trial. medRxiv. 2023;**6**(7):e2323205

[50] Chinoda S, Mutsinze A, Simms V, et al. Effectiveness of a peer-led adolescent mental health intervention on HIV virological suppression and mental health in Zimbabwe: Protocol of a cluster-randomised trial. Global Mental Health (Cambridge). 2020;**7**:e23

[51] Kurth AE, Chhun N, Cleland CM, Crespo-Fierro M, Parés-Avila JA, Lizcano JA, et al. Linguistic and cultural adaptation of a computer-based counseling program (CARE+ Spanish) to support HIV treatment adherence and risk reduction for people living with HIV/AIDS: A randomized controlled trial. Journal of Medical Internet Research. 2016;**18**:e195

[52] Lyatuu GW, Naburi H, Mwashemele S, et al. Effect of peer-mother interactive programme on prevention of mother-to-child HIV transmission outcomes among pregnant women on anti-retroviral treatment in routine healthcare in Dar es Salaam, Tanzania. PLOS Global Public Health. 2022;**2**:e0000256

[53] Jobarteh K, Shiraishi RW, Malimane I, Samo Gudo P, Decroo T, Auld AF, et al. Community ART support groups in Mozambique: The potential of patients as partners in care. PLoS One. 2016;**11**:e0166444

[54] Decroo T, Telfer B, Dores CD, White RA, Santos ND, Mkwamba A, et al. Effect of community ART groups on retention-in-care among patients on ART in Tete Province, Mozambique: A cohort study. BMJ Open. 2017;**7**:e016800

[55] Bezabhe WM, Chalmers L, Bereznicki LR, Peterson GM. Adherence to antiretroviral therapy and Virologic failure: A meta-analysis. Medicine. 2016;**95**:e3361

[56] Nachega JB, Hislop M, Nguyen H, Dowdy DW, Chaisson RE, Regensberg L, et al. Antiretroviral therapy adherence, virologic and immunologic outcomes in adolescents compared with adults in Southern Africa. Journal of Acquired Immune Deficiency Syndromes. 2009;**51**:65-71

[57] Kingsada A. Can financial incentives improve access to care? Evidence from a French experiment on specialist physicians. Social Science & Medicine. 2024;**352**:117018

[58] Lavergne MR. Financial incentives for physicians to improve health care. CMAJ: Canadian Medical Association Journal. 2017;**189**:E1505

[59] Krishnamoorthy Y, Rehman T, Sakthivel M. Effectiveness of financial incentives in achieving UNAID fast-track 90-90-90 and 95-95-95 target of HIV care continuum: A systematic review and Meta-analysis of randomized controlled trials. AIDS and Behavior. 2021;**25**:814-825

[60] Metsch LR, Feaster DJ, Gooden L, et al. Effect of patient navigation with or without financial incentives on viral suppression among hospitalized patients with HIV infection and substance use: A randomized clinical trial. JAMA. 2016;**316**:156-170

[61] Agwu AL, Yusuf HE, D'Angelo L, et al. Recruitment of youth living with HIV to optimize adherence and virologic suppression: Testing the design of

technology-based community health nursing to improve antiretroviral therapy (ART) clinical trials. JMIR Research Protocols. 2020;**9**:e23480

[62] Kalichman SC, Kalichman MO, Eaton LA. Phone-delivered intervention to improve HIV Care for Young People Living with HIV: Trial to inform implementation and utility. Journal of Acquired Immune Deficiency Syndromes. 2023;**94**:227-234

[63] Jiao K, Ma J, Lin Y, et al. Effectiveness of instant versus text messaging intervention on antiretroviral therapy adherence among men who have sex with men living with HIV. Digit Health. 2024;**10**:20552076241257447

Section 3

Advances in Antiviral Drug Development and Mechanisms

Chapter 4

Peptide-Based Fusion Inhibitors Targeting 6-HB: Resistance to HIV-1 outside of Cells

Guodong Liang, Yan Huang, Jinlin Wang, Xin Gao, Yuting Zhao, Lu Ga, Yan Zhao, Yuheng Ma, Yunfeng Xiao, Taoran Wang, Yihui Jin and Ruijuan Li

Abstract

Pathogenic viruses causing large outbreaks often contain Class I fusion proteins on their envelopes. These proteins facilitate virus-host cell membrane fusion through a common mechanism involving the N-terminal Heptad Repeat region forming a coiled-coil trimer and the C-terminal region folding back to form a six-helix bundle (6-HB). Fusion inhibitors, particularly peptide-based ones like Enfuvirtide and Albuvirtide, target the 6-HB to block membrane fusion and have been clinically approved. Researchers have always been committed to digging out more peptide-based fusion inhibitors lead candidates and better molecular mechanisms. More compound structural optimization may predominate in future research, which we believe will lay a solid foundation for improving drug performance. This chapter offers a comprehensive review of the structure and function of 6-HB, along with the latest developments in peptide-based fusion inhibitors. Our insights aim to serve as a handy guide for researchers, offering inspiration and valuable information in this field.

Keywords: HIV-1, antivirals, 6-HB, fusion inhibitors, peptide

1. Introduction

Both human health and the advancement of social civilization face considerable harm from emerging viral infectious diseases. For example, Acquired Immune Deficiency Syndrome (AIDS) is a devastating infectious disease caused by the Human Immunodeficiency Virus type 1 (HIV-1). The latest Joint United Nations Programme on HIV/AIDS (UNAIDS) reports show that there are currently 39 million AIDS patients worldwide, 29.8 million of whom are on antiretroviral treatment, 1.3 million new HIV infections in 2022, and 630,000 deaths from AIDS-related illnesses (https://thepath.unaids.org/). The "One Bug-One Drug" approach for developing antiviral agents has achieved multiple remarkable successes in the ongoing battle against viruses [1]. Yet, in recent years, the rise of drug resistance and the unforeseen devastation wrought by emerging viruses, like SARS-CoV-2, have highlighted the potential limitations of the "One Bug-One Drug" approach in tackling the escalating variety of infections caused by unidentified pathogens [2, 3]. Therefore, exploiting novel and effective antivirals is still an urgent task.

Viruses may be extensively divided into two categories: enveloped viruses and non-enveloped viruses, based on whether they possess a lipid-rich envelope external to their protein capsid [4]. As the virus matures, it acquires its envelope from the cytoplasmic or nuclear membrane of the host cell, incorporating glycosylated proteins that are crucial for facilitating viral membrane fusion [5, 6]. Fusion inhibitors work in the early phase of membrane fusion during enveloped virus infection. Fusion inhibitors block the membrane fusion of the viral envelope with the host cell membrane or endosomal membrane by inhibiting the conformational changes of the fusion protein [7]. Unlike other antiviral drugs that inhibit viral replication inside host cells, fusion inhibitors are formulated to act outside the cell, focusing on the early stages of viral replication, like viral fusion. The advantage of this approach is that the therapeutic inhibitor does not need to penetrate the cell membrane, thereby minimizing potential harmful interactions between the viral pathogen and host cells [8]. The fusion inhibitors consist mainly of peptides, antibodies, small-molecule chemicals, and so on. Our research paper is dedicated to exploring fusion inhibitors that utilize peptides as their foundation [9, 10].

2. C-peptide fusion inhibitors

2.1 Origins and mechanism

The peptide-based fusion inhibitors originated in the HIV-1 field. Generally, HIV-1 attaches to host cell membrane and envelope protein subunit gp120 then binds to the cell receptor $CD4^+$ and the co-receptor CXCR4 or CCR5, triggering transmembrane subunit gp41 conformational changes. Insertion of the gp41 N-terminus into the host cell membrane causes the C-terminal heptad repeat (CHR) region and the N-terminal heptad repeat (NHR) region to stretch into an intermediate state. Subsequently, the CHR region further interacts with the NHR region at the outside to form Six-helix bundle (6-HB) structure, which draws the viral envelope fusion with the host cell membrane, and facilitates fusion hole formation. Viral genetic material eventually enters the host cell through the fusion hole [11]. Compounds, which could inhibit antiviral activity by preventing endogenous 6-HB formation through binding with the CHR or NHR region, are generally referred to as fusion inhibitors [12, 13]. C-peptide fusion inhibitors, the most common peptide-based fusion inhibitor, sequences deriving from the gp41 CHR region or de novo designed, with the single-helix binding to gp41 NHR region, thus inhibiting 6-HB formation and exerting anti-HIV-1 ability (**Figure 1**) [14].

2.2 C-peptide modification strategies

Enfuvirtide (also known as T20) is the first listed C-peptide fusion inhibitor against HIV-1, which plays an important role in the AIDS treatment. However, in the clinical application process, T20 has shown major deficiencies in clinical application such as high level drug resistance, short half-life in vivo [15, 16]. And to date,

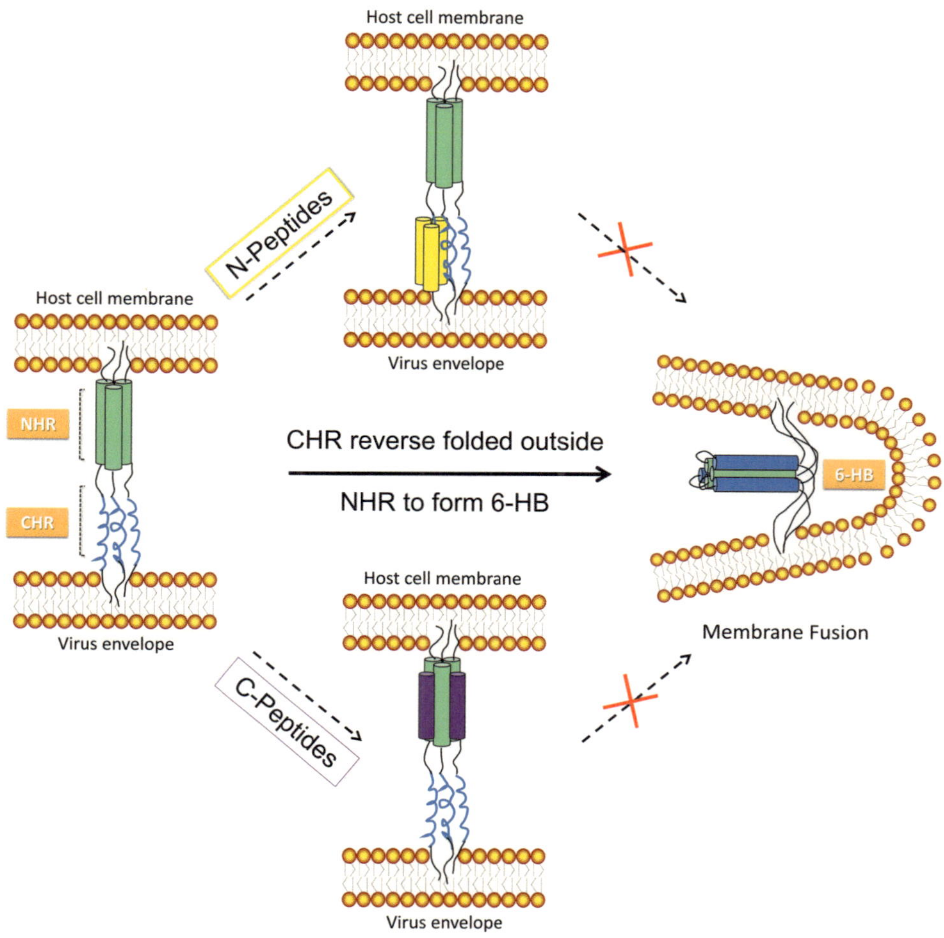

Figure 1.
The inhibitory mechanism of membrane fusion for C-peptides and N-peptides.

researchers have traveled many miles to obtain novel peptide-based fusion inhibitors, but there is still no new drug that solves the above problems [17, 18]. Here, we have summarized six latest C-peptide modification strategies in order to provide reference for future candidate development.

2.2.1 The E-K salt bridge-based modification strategy

Peptide-based fusion inhibitors bind to the target generally with α-helical conformation. But the short peptide, as current hot candidate, tends to be randomly coiled, and thus the greater entropy loss for assembly into active α-helix during interaction with the target. Salt bridges formed between side chains positioned at intervals of $(i \rightarrow i + 3)$ or $(i \rightarrow i + 4)$ (**Figure 2**) contribute favorably to the folding enthalpies, thereby compensating for the configurational entropy lost upon transitioning into an α-helix. As such, the strategy of salt bridge modification can be effectively employed for optimizing the peptide sequence.

The C34 peptide, exclusively derived from the HIV-1 gp41 CHR region [19], has demonstrated remarkable anti-HIV-1 activity, even maintaining its effectiveness

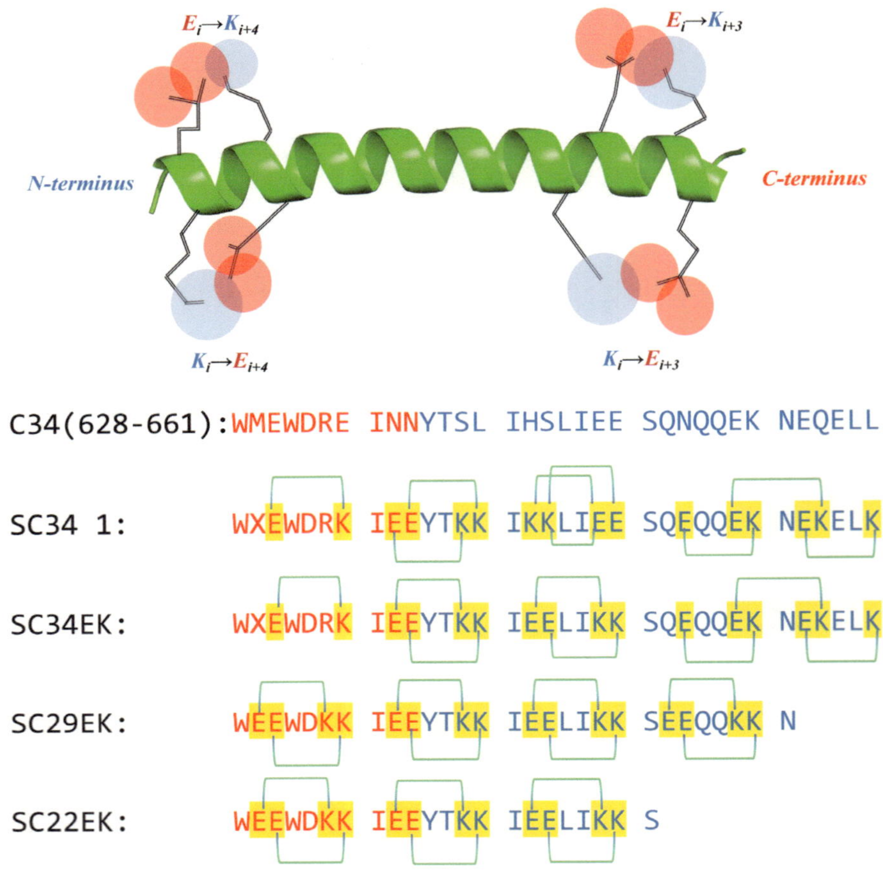

Figure 2.
The peptide sequences with E-K salt bridge (X represents norleucine amino acid residue).

against T20-resistant viral strains. However, compared to T20, C34 falls short as a candidate due to its lower solubility [20]. In 2002, Akira et al. obtained the peptide, named SC34 1, by replacing C34 residues located in the non-target binding region with hydrophilic glutamic acid (Glu) or lysine (Lys) to form the E-K salt bridge. SC34-1 not only overcame the solubility and α-helicity deficiencies of C34 but also exhibited a 10-fold increase in anti-HIV-1 activity compared to T20 [21]. Hiroki et al. further refined SC34-1 by reversing the E-K salt bridges at positions 16, 17, and 20, 21 in the sequence, resulting in SC34EK (**Figure 2**) [22]. The crystal structure of the SC34EK/target complex revealed that SC34EK adopted a standard α-helix due to the E-K salt bridges and had a propensity to form a heterologous 6-HB with the target peptide N36. The inhibitory activity of SC35EK against T20-resistant strains (including L33S, V38E, N43D, V38E/N42S) reached 0.9–4.3 nM, while T20's inhibitory activity exceeded 1000 nM.

The E-K salt bridge modification has been proven to enhance α-helix formation and anti-HIV-1 activity, even conferring the ability to inhibit T20-resistant strains. Takeshi et al. shortened the SC34EK sequence to create SC29EK (**Figure 2**) [23]. SC29EK not only inhibited HIV-1 infection at a level comparable to SC34EK, but also blocked the replication of T20-resistant strains (EC_{50} = 2.7–4.1 nM) and maintained antiviral activity even in the presence of 50% serum concentrations. Hiroki et al. further truncated SC29EK to 22 peptide, named SC22EK (**Figure 2**) [24]. SC22EK currently stands as the shortest peptide employing the E-K salt bridge strategy. Experimental results indicated that SC22EK could suppress the C34-resistant strain (although data on T20-resistant strains was not available) and maintained significant anti-HIV-1 activity and high binding affinity. Therefore, designing peptides based on the E-K salt bridge strategy is a highly feasible approach that improves solubility, maintains the α-helix active conformation, and ultimately demonstrates potential inhibitory activity against the drug-resistant strains [25].

2.2.2 The stapled peptide-based modification strategy

Researchers have recognized that peptides derived directly from the natural sequences of fusion proteins often bind to their targets in secondary structures such as α-helices [26–28]. However, a significant challenge is that many peptide fragments are unable to form stable secondary structures and are prone to hydrolysis by peptidases, leading to reduced activity and bioavailability [29]. Fixation of the peptide helical structure by chemical modification has been shown to solve the above problems (**Figure 3**). In 2000, Verdine et al. introduced a method to stabilize the α-helical structure known as "Stapled Peptide." This method utilizes carbon-carbon bonds as a scaffold to reinforce the helical conformation of the peptide, thereby enhancing its stability and potentially improving its bioactivity and resistance to enzymatic degradation [30]. By employing such strategies, researchers can develop more effective and durable peptide-based therapies for various diseases, including HIV-1.

Inspired by the stapled modification strategy, Bird et al. obtained T20-1 and T20-2 by introducing the conformational stapled backbone at the *(i, i + 4)* site in T20 sequence (**Figure 4**) [31]. Their findings revealed that as the number of stapled backbones increased, the resistance to enzymes and anti-HIV activity of T20 also enhanced. Building on this, Meng et al. chose T2635, containing both the pocket binding domain (PBD) sequence and the helix binding domain (HBD) sequence, as a template for designing short-peptide fusion inhibitors. They truncated T2635 into a 22-mer peptide, designated CP22, by removing its N-terminal T-T motif, the PBD region, and the PBD downstream sequence from residues Ala-11 to Arg-16.

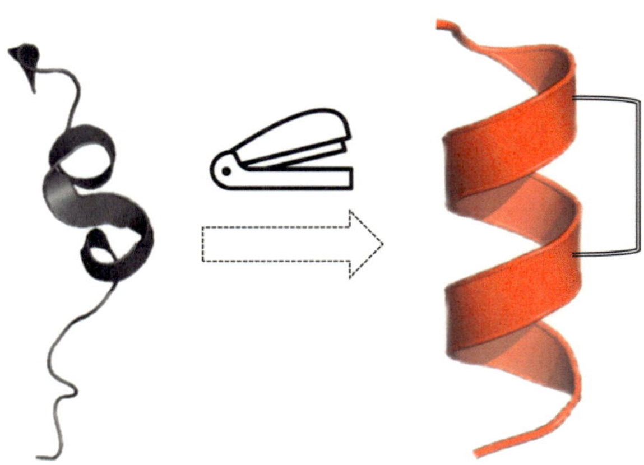

Figure 3.
The schematic diagram of stapled modification strategy.

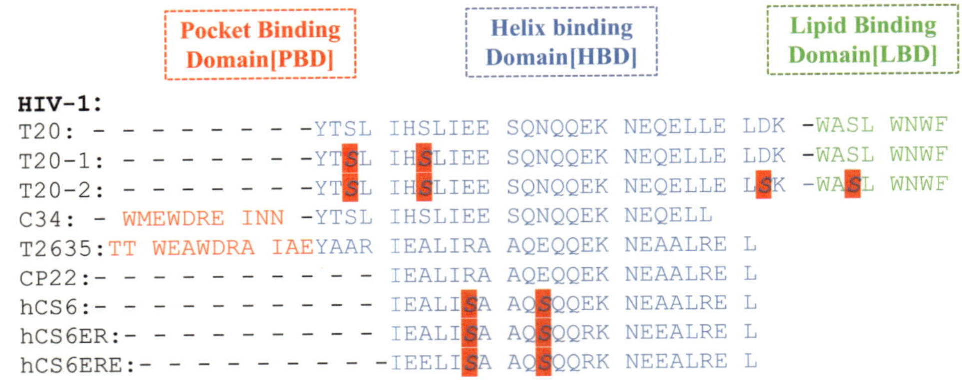

Figure 4.
Schematic diagram of stapled peptides (S represents the stapled site).

Subsequently, they applied cysteine or homocysteine alkylation to CP22, yielding the *m*-xylene thioether stapled short peptides hCS6, hCS6RE, and hCS6ERE (**Figure 4**). The stapled peptides had higher helicity than the linear peptides and exhibited improved metabolic stability over T20. Among stapled peptides, hCS6ERE exhibited 11 nM inhibitory activity against HIV-1_{IIIB} strain, nearly 3-fold higher than T20, and 15.2 nM inhibitory activity against HIV-1_{Bal} strain comparable to T20. Moreover, hCS6ERE was able to inhibit T20-resistant HIV-1 strains and T2635-resistant HIV-1 strains in combination with peptide inhibitor HP23 [32]. The stapled modification strategy has proven its versatility not only in the development of HIV-1 peptide inhibitors but also in the design of short-peptide inhibitors for other viruses with similar membrane fusion mechanisms. In 2018, Wang et al. successfully applied this strategy to design peptides targeting the N-terminal heptad repeat (NHR) region in the Middle East Respiratory Syndrome Coronavirus (MERS-CoV) S protein. The resulting peptide, P21S10, demonstrated effective inhibition of MERS-CoV infection and spike protein-mediated cell-cell fusion [33]. P21S10 exhibited stronger metabolic stability in vitro and superior pharmacokinetic properties compared to P21, which lacked a stapled backbone. Therefore, the stapled peptide strategy represents another effective approach to enhance the inhibitory activity and stability of novel fusion inhibitors. It enables the development of short peptides that can inhibit drug-resistant strains, facilitating advancements in drug development for HIV-1 and potentially other diseases.

2.2.3 The strategy for "M-T hook" introduction at the peptide N-terminus

The information provided describes an investigation by He et al. into the upstream motif of the C-terminal heptad repeat (CHR) peptide binding domain (PBD) region. They designed a peptide, CP621-652, that contains the "QIWNNMT" sequence at positions 621–627 of the CHR. This peptide interacts with a target peptide from the N-terminal heptad repeat (NHR) region to form a stable six-helix bundle (6-HB) structure. The "M-T hook" structure is a specific conformation formed by the conserved residues Met-626 and Thr-627 within the "QIWNNMT" sequence. Although most of the residues in this sequence are disordered in the electron density, Met-626 and Thr-627 fold into a quasi-hook shape that stabilizes the 6-HB structure (**Figure 5**). In this structure, Thr-627 alters the orientation of the peptide chain and

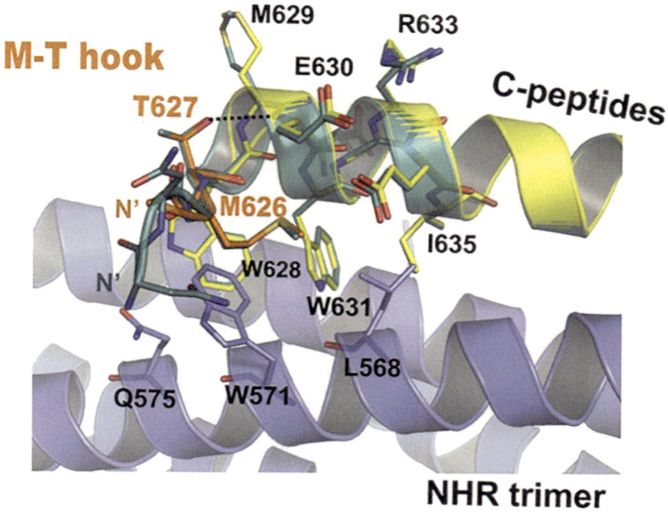

Figure 5.
Crystal structure of the "M-T Hook" structure [34].

positions Met-626 on top of a hydrophobic pocket. The side chain of Met-626 acts as a cover for the hydrophobic pocket, stabilizing the interaction between the pocket and the pocket-binding domain. This stabilization contributes to the overall strength and stability of the 6-HB structure, making CP621-652 a more effective inhibitor of viral fusion than peptides lacking the "QIWNNMT" sequence [33–35].

The research by He et al. and Chong et al. highlights the potential of the "M-T Hook" structure in optimizing HIV-1 fusion inhibitors. By mutating 11 residues in the CP621-652 peptide, He et al. obtained a novel 32-amino acid HIV-1 fusion inhibitor called CP32M. This peptide, which retains the "M-T Hook" structure, forms stable 6-HB complexes with the NHR region. CP32M can efficiently inhibit infection by several well-characterized T20-resistant viruses that carry an L33S point mutation or I37Q/V38Q, I37Q/V38M, and I37V/V38T double mutations; in sharp contrast, T20 had no inhibitory activity at a concentration as high as 750 nM [36]. Furthermore, Chong et al. obtained MT-C34 and MT-SFT by introducing "M-T Hook" at the N-terminus of C34 and Sifuvirtide, which showed stronger antiviral ability, and even the ability against T20-resistant strains [37]. Therefore, the "M-T Hook" structural modification strategy is an effective method to optimize the lead peptide, which keeps the peptide with highly antiviral activity, and may facilitate further sequence shortening. They also introduced the "M-T Hook" at the N-terminal of shorter peptides SC29EK and SC22EK, obtaining MT-SC29EK and MT-SC22EK, which retained high potency against T20- and SC29EK-resistant viruses (**Figure 6**) [38]. Based on the structural basis of MT-SC22EK, Chong et al. finally obtained a short peptide HP23 with 23 amino acid residues, which even exhibited picomolar anti-HIV-1 activity [39]. HP23 consists of "M-T Hook" structure, all PDB region and partial HBD region, tightly targeting the N-trimer of HIV-1 gp41 (**Figure 6**) [40]. HP23 was highly active in the inhibition of diverse HIV-1 subtypes, including T20 and MT-SC22EK-resistant HIV-1 mutants, and it exhibited a high genetic barrier to the development of resistance. The "M-T Hook" structure indeed provides more opportunities for peptides to interact with their targets and combat T20-resistant strains of HIV-1. This structural modification strategy has shown promising results in optimizing HIV-1 fusion

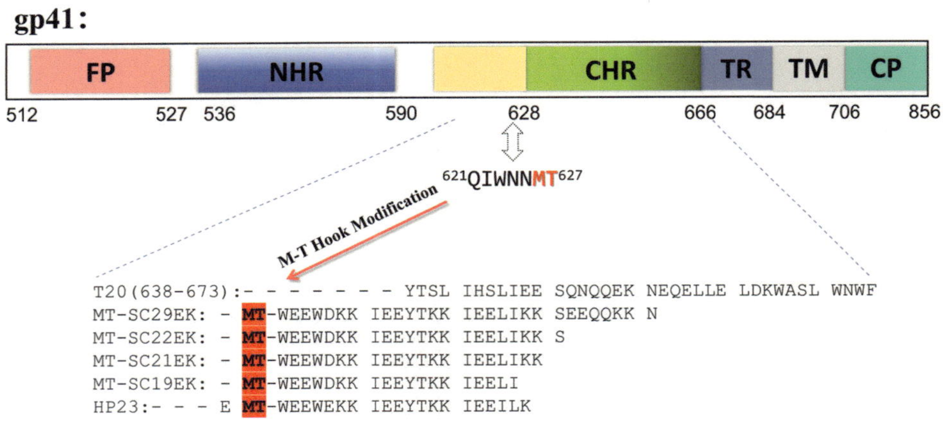

Figure 6.
The peptide sequences containing "M-T Hook" portion.

inhibitors and enhancing their antiviral activity. Therefore, peptides incorporating the "M-T Hook" structure are expected to be further developed and tested as potential drug candidates for the treatment of HIV-1 infection.

2.2.4 The strategy for "IDL tail" introduction at the peptide C-terminus

It is well known that peptides containing "M-T Hook" structure in N-terminus showed anti-HIV-1, and even favored shorter sequences, so is it possible to introduce a particular structure at peptide C-terminus to obtain alternative novel short-peptide inhibitors? Guidance based on this question, researchers have identified another hook structure called the "IDL Tail" in the C-terminus of peptides. This structure is composed of isoleucine (Ile), aspartate (Asp), and leucine (Leu) residues and has been shown to interact with the NHR trimer of HIV-1 gp41 in a specific way. In the "IDL Tail" structure (**Figure 7**), the Ile and Leu hydrophobic side chains are oriented toward the NHR trimer and bind to the hydrophobic residues Leu545 and Val549. The Asp hydrophilic side chain targets the NHR through forming a salt bridge with the Asn553 side chain. Additionally, the Gln653 and Gln649 residues can form hydrogen bonds upstream of the "IDL Tail," which further stabilize its structure.

Inspired by the gp41-derived MT hook, Yun et al. synthesized the first short peptide against HIV-1, called CP-IDL, containing "IDL Tail" (**Figure 8**) [41]. The original CP peptide has low inhibitory activities against HIV-1 clinical strains, with IC_{50} of 281 and 207 nM, respectively, while CP-IDL showed the highest potency with increase of 109- and 55-fold, respectively. Also, CP-IDL could inhibit infection of all these T2635 or T20-resistant strains, which are much more potent than CP or T20. Furthermore, Chong et al. identified a shorter peptide [42], HP23, but found that it became ineffective against HIV-1 strains with the E49K mutation in the gp41 NHR region. However, by extending the C-terminus of HP23 with the "IDL Tail" structure, they created HP23-E6-IDL (**Figure 8**), which ameliorated the resistance to HP23 and showed increased inhibitory efficacy against HIV-1 strains and HP23-resistant mutants [43]. Compared to HP23, HP23-E6-IDL showed 2-fold to 16-fold increase in inhibitory efficacy against HIV-1 strains, and 12-fold increase in efficacy against HP23-resistant mutants. Subsequently, Su et al. synthesized other peptides, WQ-IDL and MT-WQ-IDL (**Figure 8**), by adding the "IDL Tail" structure and found that they showed more

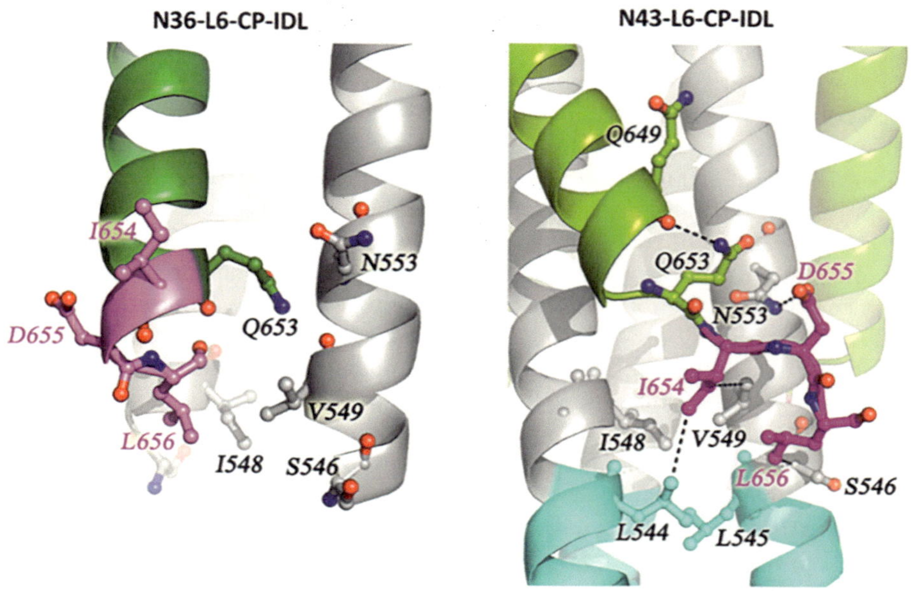

Figure 7.
Crystal structure of the "IDL Tail" structure [41].

```
T20(638-673):- - - - - - - - YTSL IHSLIEE SQNQQEK NEQELLE LDK -WASL WNWF
CP:- - - - - - - WEEWDKK IEE -YTKK IEELIKK SQNQQ
CP-IDL:- - - - - WEEWDKK IEE -YTKK IEELIKK SQNQQ-IDL
HP23-E6-IDL:E-MT-WEEWERK IEE -YTKK IEEILKK SQNQQ-IDL
YIK:- - - - E-MT-WEEWEKK IEE -YIKK IEEILKK SQNOQ-IDL
WQ-IDI:- - - - - WEEWDKK IEE -YTKK IEELIKK SQNQQ-IDL
MT-WQ-IDL:- - MT-WEEWDKK IEE -YTKK IEELIKK SQNQQ-IDL
```

IDL Tail Modification

Figure 8.
The peptide sequences containing "IDL Tail" portion.

potent activities than T20 in inhibiting HIV-1_{IIIB} infection [44]. In a later study, Su et al. introduced a mutation (T639I) into HP23-E6-IDL to generate the peptide YIK, which effectively inhibited HIV-1 infection and had a longer half-life [45]. While the peptides obtained using this strategy have not been fully investigated for their ability to inhibit T20-resistant strains, the results suggest that adding non-helical tails at the C-terminus may be a valid and universal strategy to improve the antiviral potency of C-peptide fusion inhibitors. As with the "M-T Hook" structure, further research and testing will be needed to evaluate the potential of "IDL Tail"-containing peptides as drug candidates for the treatment of HIV-1 infection.

2.2.5 The specific small-molecule conjugation strategy

We have known that, unlike peptides, small-molecule inhibitors boast cost-effectiveness and robust stability, rendering them highly favorable for pharmaceutical development [46, 47]. Within the realm of anti-HIV-1 fusion inhibitors, two small molecules—NB-2 and A12—have garnered attention for their micromolar-level activity against HIV-1 by targeting the PBD (Pocket Binding Domain) region of gp41 [20]. Notably, C34, a peptide harboring the PBD sequence, exhibits binding affinity toward the NHR (N-terminal Heptad Repeat) hydrophobic pocket, aligning with the specific target site of these small molecules [48]. Researchers have innovatively substituted the PBD segment of C34 with small molecules, thereby crafting small molecule-peptide conjugates (**Figure 9**). These conjugates harness a synergistic binding mechanism, where the small molecule and peptide portions lock onto distinct NHR regions. Wang et al. demonstrated this by excising the PBD portion of C34 to yield the peptide P26, and subsequently appending either A12 or NB-2 to the N-terminus of P26 (**Figure 10**) [49]. HIV-1 envelope protein-mediated cell-cell fusion assays have validated the superiority of these conjugates, exhibiting heightened inhibitory activity compared to their individual components or P26 alone. Remarkably, they effectively neutralized both T20-sensitive and T20-resistant HIV-1 strains, indicating that this specific conjugation strategy not only enhances antiviral efficacy but also exhibits drug resistance tolerance.

Saponins, a class of bioactive natural compounds primarily synthesized by plants as a defense mechanism against pathogens and herbivores, have demonstrated extensive antiviral properties. Notably, several pentacyclic triterpene saponins, including chikusetsusaponin IVa and glycyrrhizin, have exhibited broad antiviral activities [50]. Wang et al. synthesized alternative small molecule-peptide conjugates by linking saponin compounds to P26 *via* "Click Chemistry" (**Figure 11**) [33]. In this process, saponin compounds were linked to the P26 peptide, resulting in conjugates that exhibited remarkable anti-HIV-1 activity, enhanced in vivo metabolic stability, and potent inhibitory effects against T20-resistant strains. Building on this success, our team further refined the concept by successfully synthesizing indole derivative-peptide conjugates. These conjugates featured a truncated peptide covalently attached to a gp41-targeting indole compound, once again utilizing "Click Chemistry" for efficient linkage. Remarkably, the short peptide portion in these conjugates could be shortened to just 19 amino acid residues [39]. Among these conjugates, the Indole-T26 and

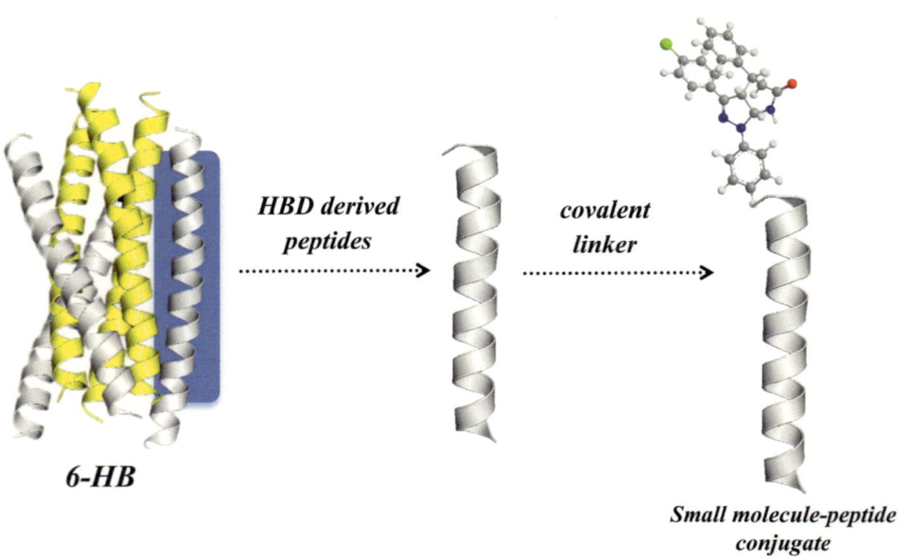

Figure 9.
The schematic diagram of specific small-molecule and peptide conjugate.

Specific small molecules:

NB-2: N-(4-carboxy-3-hydroxyphenyl)-2,5-dimethylpyrrole

A12: N-(3-carboxy-4-hydroxyphenyl)-2,5-dimethylpyrrole

Peptides:

C34:- - -WMEWDRE INNYTSL IHSLIEE SQNQQEK NEQELL

P26:- - - - - - - NNYTSL IHSLIEE SQNQQEK NEQELL

Specific small molecule-peptide conjugates:

Npc-P26: **Npc**-NNYTSL IHSLIEE SQNQQEK NEQELL

Apc-P26: **Apc**-NNYTSL IHSLIEE SQNQQEK NEQELL

Noc-P26: **Noc**-NNYTSL IHSLIEE SQNQQEK NEQELL

Aoc-P26: **Aoc**-NNYTSL IHSLIEE SQNQQEK NEQELL

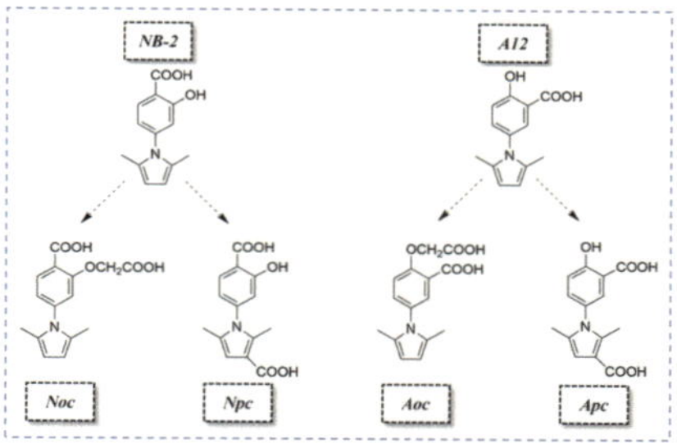

Figure 10.
The schematic of pyrrole-derived small molecule-peptide conjugate.

Specific small molecules:

BA:Betulinic acid; UA:Ursolic acid; OA:Oleanolic acid

Peptides:

C34:WMEWDRE INNYTSL IHSLIEE SQNQQEK NEQELL

P26:- - - -NNYTSL IHSLIEE SQNQQEK NEQELL

Specific small molecule-peptide conjugates:

BA-P26: - **BA**-NNYTSL IHSLIEE SQNQQEK NEQELL

UA-P26: - **UA**-NNYTSL IHSLIEE SQNQQEK NEQELL

OA-P26: - **OA**-NNYTSL IHSLIEE SQNQQEK NEQELL

P26-BA: - - -NNYTSL IHSLIEE SQNQQEK NEQELL-**BA**

P26-UA: - - -NNYTSL IHSLIEE SQNQQEK NEQELL-**UA**

P26-OA: - - -NNYTSL IHSLIEE SQNQQEK NEQELL-**OA**

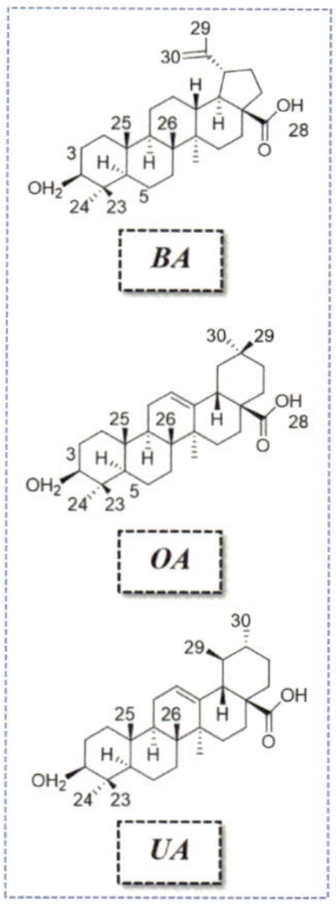

Figure 11.
The schematic of saponins-derived small molecule-peptide conjugate.

Indole-T22 inhibited HIV-1 Env-mediated cell-cell fusion and HIV-1_{NL4-3} infection at low nanomolar levels, rivaling the potency of the T20.

In summary, the specific small-molecule peptide conjugation strategy offers a novel and effective approach to truncating long peptides into compact fragments while unlocking their therapeutic potential through coupling with specific small molecules. This innovative method holds promise as a means to address the limitations of both small molecules and long peptides by combining their respective advantages and mitigating their disadvantages. The resulting conjugates exhibit a robust synergistic effect, enhancing antiviral activity and metabolic stability, which could pave the way for the development of more potent and resilient therapeutic agents against HIV-1 and other viral infections.

2.2.6 The lipid small molecule conjugation strategy

The strategy of conjugating specific small molecules to the N-terminus of CHR-derived peptides, which bind to the NHR hydrophobic pocket domain, has been shown to enhance anti-HIV-1 activity and address issues of viral drug resistance. Additionally, researchers have identified other types of small molecules, such as cholesterol and fatty acids, that can substitute for the LBD portion in CHR-derived peptide sequences. These molecules facilitate the anchoring of peptide portion to the cell membrane, thereby increasing target region concentration (**Figure 12**) [51–55]. These small molecules could not specifically recognize NHR region, but rather enhance anti-HIV-1 capacity by enriching peptide concentrations in the membrane fusion region through non-specific effects such as lipophilicity, and are therefore considered "lipid-small molecule."

The integration of fatty acids into peptide scaffolds has emerged as a promising strategy for optimizing peptide-based fusion inhibitors, as demonstrated by Wexler's early findings that fatty acid incorporation enhances antiviral activity by mimicking the LBD [56–61]. Similarly, Hollmann et al. successfully linked cholesterol to the C34 sequence, resulting in a significant boost in anti-HIV-1 activity [58]. In 2016, Chong et al. synthesized a series of lipopeptides, among which LP-11, a fatty acid-conjugated lipopeptide comprising only 23 residues (**Figure 13**), exhibited potent and broad inhibitory activity against a diverse array of HIV-1 isolates and clinically resistant mutants. On this basis, Chong et al. further refined their approach by developing LP-19, a novel lipopeptide inhibitor with 23 residues (**Figure 13**), which incorporated multiple design strategies, including the M-T hook structure, partial HIV-2 sequences, and a membrane-anchoring lipid tail [62]. In vitro studies showed that T20, LP-11, and LP-19 inhibited T20-resistant mutants with mean IC50 values of 1804, 0.37, and 0.17 nM, respectively. Notably, LP-19 displayed significantly increased

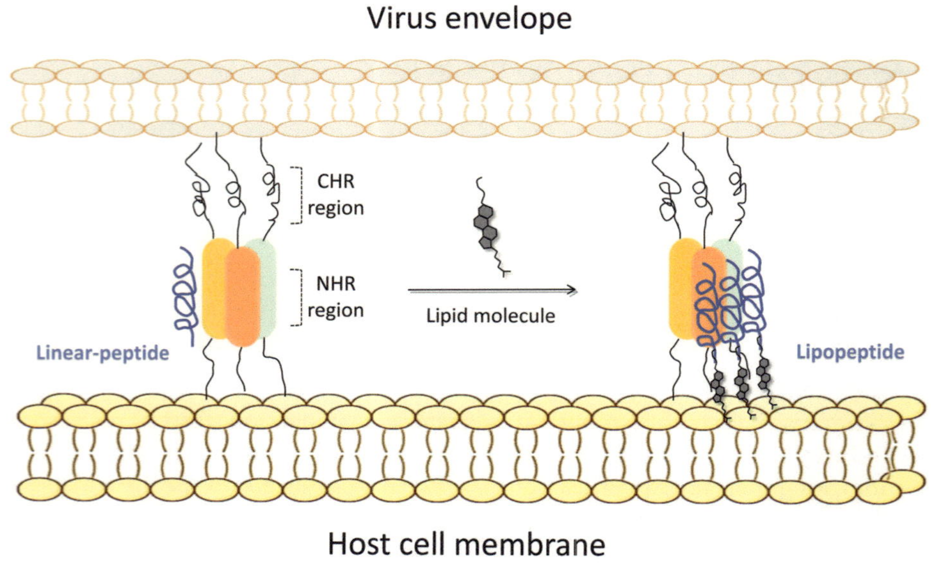

Figure 12.
Putative mode of action of HIV-1 lipopeptides. The NHR domain is shown in the color column, the CHR domain is shown in the black spiral line, the non-lipopeptide is shown in the blue spiral line, and the lipopeptide is shown in the blue spiral line plus lipid molecule tail.

Non-specific small molecule:

Cholesterol

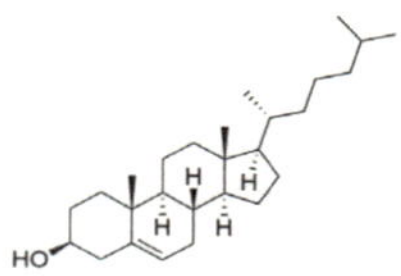

Palmitic acid(C16)

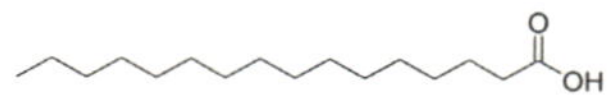

Peptides:

C34: - - -WMEWDRE INNYTSL IHSLIEE SQNQQEK NEQELL
HP23:- - -WEEWEKK IEEYTKK IEEILK

Non-specific small molecule-peptide conjugates:

C34-chol: WMEWDRE INNYTSL IHSLIEE SQNQQEK NEQELL-**Chol**
LP-11: EMTWEEWEKK IEEYTKK IEEILK-**C16**
LP-19: EMTWEEWEKK VEELEKK IEELLK-**C16**

Figure 13.
The sequences of lipid-small molecule-peptide conjugate (Cholesterol, Palmitic acid).

potency against both T20- and HP23-resistant viruses. In summary, LP-19 represents a promising candidate for clinical application development due to its potent antiviral activity, broad spectrum of activity, and resistance-breaking potential. This lipopeptide inhibitor holds significant promise for addressing the challenges posed by drug-resistant HIV-1 variants and improving the therapeutic options available for HIV-infected patients.

In addition, we venture to speculate whether it is possible to use both specific and non-specific small molecules in combination with peptide couples. This approach, which encapsulates the targeting specificity of specific small molecules with the membrane-targeting ability of non-specific small molecules, has the potential to overcome the limitations of the above conjugates, providing a versatile and promising strategy for the development of potent antiviral agents.

3. N-peptide fusion inhibitors

3.1 Origins and mechanism

The membrane fusion process of class I viruses involves a complex interplay between the N-terminal heptad repeat (NHR) and C-terminal heptad repeat (CHR) regions. During this process, the NHR regions undergo allosteric changes to form the N-trimer structural core. Subsequently, the CHR regions fold with the N-trimer to create a six-helix bundle (6-HB) structural domain. This 6-HB formation is crucial for viral fusion and entry into host cells. Current research has revealed that peptides sourced from the NHR domain are crucial for impeding the natural development of 6-HB by creating N-trimer mimetic structures that selectively attach to the CHR domain (**Figure 1**) [63]. Building on the previous point, N-peptides originating from the NHR sequences of class I viruses like HIV, MERS-CoV, and EBOV (Ebola Virus) have effectively modified the active conformation of the N-trimer and even demonstrated antiviral properties [12, 64–67]. Consequently, the N-trimer functions as the essential foundation of viral fusion, and its significance in the fusion mechanism has paved the way for the identification of N-peptide lead compounds. These compounds directly reshape the native N-trimer or construct N-trimer mimics utilizing biochemical techniques. These discoveries have significant implications for the development of antiviral therapies targeting class I viruses, as they provide a potential means to disrupt the viral fusion process and prevent viral entry into host cells.

3.2 Two basic approaches to modify N-peptides

As previously stated, the two principal methods for modifying N-peptides are either mutating particular positions in the peptide sequences or integrating supplementary proteins or peptides into the peptide sequences. Each of these approaches aims to enhance the stability and inhibitory activity of the N-peptides. In the first approach, mutational modification involves altering specific amino acids in the peptide sequence based on the structure and function of the N-trimer molecule and the pattern of triple-helix formation. This can bolster the N-peptide's spatial configuration stability and its capacity to interact with the target location, thereby augmenting its inhibitory effectiveness. As an example, Bewley et al. engineered $N36_{Mut(e,g)}$ through the substitution of nine amino acids at the specified (e.g.) site of N36. This mutant peptide exhibited increased inhibitory activity with a concentration of 308 nanomolar and functions by blocking the formation of endogenous 6-HB with the natural N-trimer [68]. The second approach involves embedding accessory proteins or peptides within the sequence to enhance the ability to assemble triple-helix structures. This can overcome the disadvantages of self-polymerization sediment and allow the novel N-peptides to form N-trimer mimics under suitable solution or physiological conditions. Debra et al. combined the instrumental peptide GCN4-pIQI' with N36, N23, and N17 in the NHR region of HIV-1 gp41 to construct N-peptides' chimeric variants (**Figure 14**). These chimeric peptides exhibited nanomolar levels of inhibitory activity, demonstrating the effectiveness of this approach in enhancing antiviral activity. Overall, both approaches have shown promise in improving the inhibitory activity of N-peptides against HIV-1.

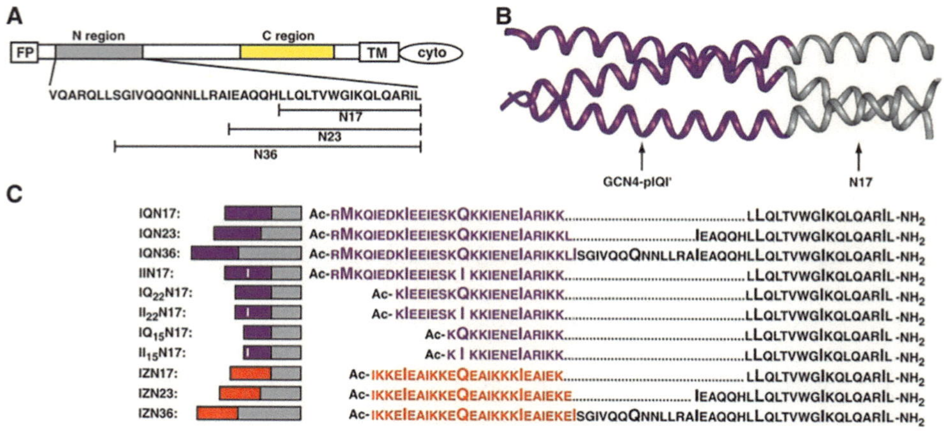

Figure 14.
The architecture of HIV-1 gp41 and the design of chimeric N peptides. (A) An illustrative depiction of the primary structural arrangement of HIV-1 gp41. (B) Model of IQN17. (C) The sequence composition of the chimeric N-peptide [12].

3.3 The isopeptide bond bundling triple-helix for designing N-peptides

3.3.1 The creation of isopeptide linkages by incorporating tool peptides into the N-peptides

An isopeptide bond is a special kind of amide bond present in proteins or peptides, and it is defined by the inclusion of at least one amino or carboxyl side chain that is not located at the alpha position. This bond has been found to play a crucial role in stabilizing protein structures, as demonstrated by Kang et al. in their study of the Gram-positive bacterial pilus Spy0128 structure in 2007 [69]. Howarth's team further investigated the mechanism of isopeptide bond formation and identified Lysine (Lys), Asparagine (Asn), Aspartic acid (Asp), and Glutamate (Glu) as key amino acids involved in this process [70–72]. The formation of isopeptide bonds can confer several beneficial characteristics to remodeled proteins or peptides, including chemical stability and protease stability [73]. Given these properties, the introduction of isopeptide bonds in the design of N-trimer mimics is a theoretically promising approach. By embedding isopeptide bonds within the supercoil framework, it might be feasible to create sturdy N-trimer imitations that display resistance to both chemical degradation and protease activity. This could lead to the development of more effective antiviral therapies that target the viral fusion process and prevent viral entry into host cells.

Initially, Lai's team engineered two man-made peptides, referred to as 3HR and 4HR, with their sequences devised in accordance with the following principles (**Figure 15**): (i) By incorporating Isoleucine (Ile) residues at the (a, d) locations within the sequence, the peptides are enabled to autonomously assemble into a trimeric configuration [75]; (ii) The Glutamine (Gln) residues at the (b, c, f) positions within the sequence are utilized to enhance solubility; (iii) Arginine (Arg) and Glutamate (Glu) residues at the (g, e) position stabilize the trimer structure by electrostatic interaction in the inter-helical side chains; (iv) It is worth noting that alterations have been made to the *(g, e)* site in the second heptad, where a Lysine (Lys) residue and a Glutamic acid (Glu) residue, which carries a benzyl thioester (SBn) side chain, have been introduced. As a result, the Glu carboxyl group located at the (e) position of the n-helix has the potential to react with the Lys amino group at the (g') position of the neighboring n + 1-helix through an acyl transfer process, leading to the formation of an inter-helical isopeptide bond. To enhance the acyl transfer reaction, the Glutamine (Gln) at the (b, c) site in the second heptad has been swapped out for a Histidine (His) residue [76, 77]. Subsequent to the acyl transfer reaction taking place, the resultant trimers that were covalently stabilized were acquired and named $(3HRN23)_3$ and $(4HRN23)_3$. To one's astonishment, the trimers $(3HRN23)_3$ and $(4HRN23)_3$ displayed a high level of potential in inhibiting HIV-1 fusion, outperforming unstructured N-peptide monomers by a considerable margin. Concurrently, the N-trimer mimics, due to the presence of an isopeptide bond, exhibit exceptional resistance, allowing them to endure both thermal and chemical denaturation. Consequently, the integration of isopeptide bonds in the design of N-trimer mimics can be an effective means of establishing the spatial arrangement of various NHR segments and may even boost the inhibitory capabilities of N-peptides. This approach has the potential to lead to the development of more effective antiviral therapies that target the HIV-1 fusion process and prevent viral entry into host cells [78].

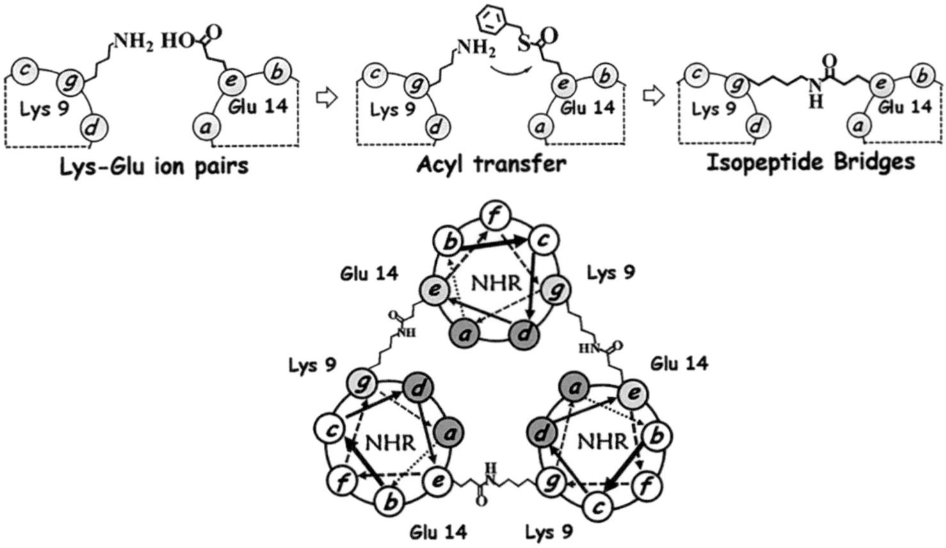

Figure 15.
A schematic depiction showcasing the generation of isopeptide bonds via an acyl transfer reaction occurring between helices, accompanied by a helical wheel representation of the N-terminal helical regions (NHRs) [74].

3.3.2 Creating isopeptide bonds via precise, location-specific mutations within the N-peptides

As has been noted, the primary approaches currently utilized for modifying N-peptides chiefly involve making targeted mutations at specific locations and integrating additional proteins or peptides. Lai's research group has revealed that the peptide is capable of being linked by isopeptide bonds after the introduction of chimeric accessory peptides. Can isopeptide bonds be formed directly after introducing mutations at key sites in the natural sequence in order to stabilize the trimeric coiled-coil configuration? Certainly, the response is in the affirmative. By employing site-directed mutagenesis on the pivotal N36 sequence found in the HIV-1 NHR region, Lai was able to create N36 mutants such as N36M, N36MEK1, and N36MEK2. These mutants exhibit the capability to autonomously form trimeric coiled coils, and this is achieved without the requirement for chimeric auxiliary proteins or peptide chains [79]. Based on the sequence of N36, the 6th residue Gln at the *(g)* position and the 11th residue Leucine (Leu) at the *(e)* position were further substituted by Lys and Glu (SBn), respectively, to form isopeptide bonds *via* an inter-helical acyl transfer reaction in coiled coil. These isopeptide bond-stabilized N-trimer mimics, $(N36M)_3$, $(N36MEK1)_3$, $(N36MEK2)_3$, exhibited potent inhibitory activities against HIV-1 fusion and infection when interacting with the ligand C34. In comparison to the commercially available Enfuvirtide, $(N36M)_3$ shows a remarkably higher level of metabolic stability when exposed to proteinase K solution, liver and kidney homogenates, and rat plasma [80]. This suggests that the isopeptide bond-stabilized N-trimer mimics have the potential to be more effective and stable antiviral therapies than existing treatments. Our team achieved artificial N-peptides using computer-aided drug design based on isopeptide bond construction (**Figure 16**). The most active compound, IZNP02QE, surpassed the positive control by demonstrating remarkable nanomolar-level inhibitory activity against HIV-1 [81].

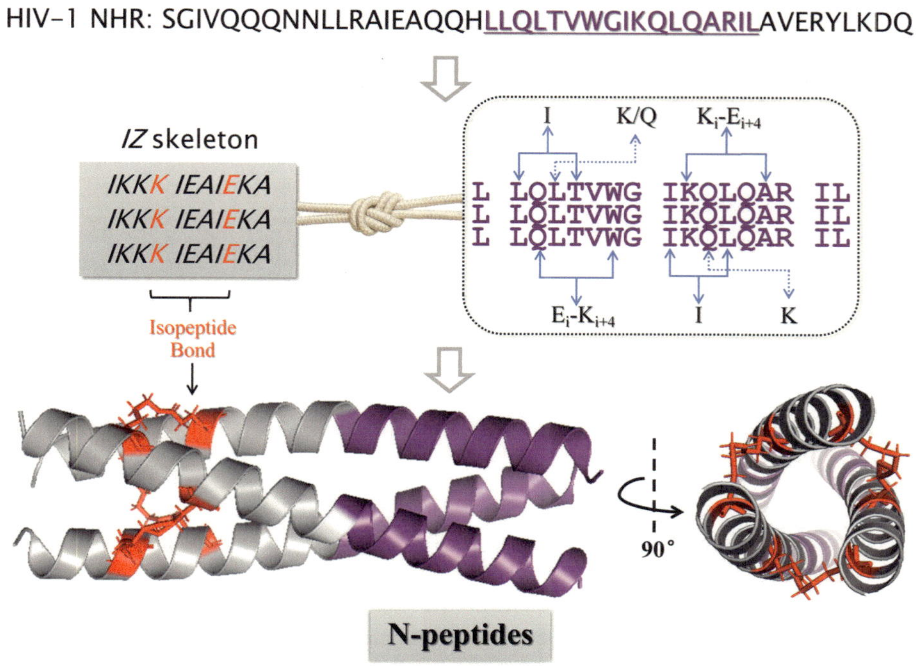

Figure 16.
The schematic N-peptide design for constructing isopeptide bonds based on site-specific mutations [81].

3.4 Breakthrough for designing broad-spectrum N-peptide inhibitors by isopeptide bond bundling triple-helix

Theoretically, for N-peptides to possess broad-spectrum antiviral activity, two essential prerequisites must be met: first, they must adopt a spatial conformation that is compatible with binding to the CHR (C-terminal heptad repeat) region of the viral envelope glycoprotein. Second, they must possess a sequence that, while potentially distinct from the natural NHR (N-terminal heptad repeat) region, still retains the ability to interact with the CHR domain in a spatially favorable manner. By utilizing the guidelines for constructing trimeric coiled coils and the mechanisms behind the creation of isopeptide bonds, N-peptides can be designed to be held together in a specific spatial arrangement by isopeptide bonds, resulting in the development of more stable imitations of N-trimers. These stabilized N-peptides, despite having sequences that differ from the natural NHR region, maintain interaction sites with the CHR domain and are capable of preventing viral membrane fusion. The distinct sequences of these covalently stabilized N-peptides may contribute to their broad-spectrum antiviral properties.

Wang et al. applied the coiled-coil design concept to modify N36 into N1G, followed by the incorporation of an isopeptide bond through an acyl transfer process, which led to the creation of the engineered peptide N3G. The results from the antiviral activity assessments indicated that N3G possesses an exceptionally broad antiviral spectrum, showing potent activity against HIV-1, MERS-CoV, the human pathogenic coronavirus OC43 (HCoV-OC43), and SARS-CoV-2 (**Figure 17**) [82]. These research findings broke through two significant challenges by constructing N-trimer

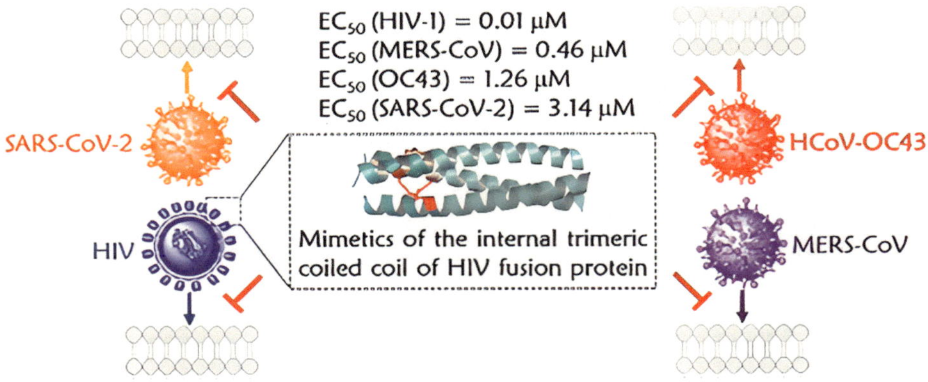

Figure 17.
The coiled-coil peptide against HIV-1 and Human β-Coronavirus infection [82].

supercoiling structure: (i) N-peptides exert high inhibitory activity against Human β-Coronavirus for the first time; (ii) N-peptides present broad-spectrum antiviral activity, breaking through virus species. Coronaviruses can infect host cells through plasma membrane pathway and endosomal pathway [83], while peptides are generally unable to enter the endosomes to exert inhibitory activity. Saskia et al. have disclosed that synthetic coiled coils, incorporating positively charged residues, are capable of traversing cellular membranes [84]. The mode of action for this coiled coil is presumably similar to that of cell-penetrating peptides (CPPs), in which the arginine (Arg) residues of CPPs strongly bind to acidic protein domains, sulfated glycans, and the hydrophilic head groups of membrane phospholipids present on the cell surface. This binding subsequently initiates the process of endocytosis [85]. Due to its coiled-coil configuration that features positively charged arginine (Arg) and lysine (Lys) residues, N3G is apt to interact with negatively charged molecular entities on the cell membrane's exterior. Such an interaction may prompt endocytosis and hinder the fusion of viral membranes within the endosome, consequently showing promise as an inhibitor against coronaviruses. In terms of its wide-ranging antiviral capabilities across different virus types, N3G undergoes a process of three-dimensional folding and self-assembly, ultimately forming an N-trimer that contains binding sites characterized by strong affinity. N3G decreases the degree of conformational entropy loss when binding to the CHR region, allowing it to create heterologous 6-HB (six-helix bundle) complexes with the CHR regions of multiple viruses via non-specific hydrophobic interactions. As a result, N3G demonstrates broad-spectrum antiviral activity.

4. Conclusion

The high pathogenicity and mutation susceptibility of viruses have driven researchers to continuously seek novel fusion inhibitors. The approval of peptide-based fusion inhibitors such as Enfuvirtide by the U.S. Food and Drug Administration (FDA) and Albuvirtide by the National Medical Products Administration (NMPA, previously known as CFDA) has paved the way for antiviral drug research [86]. Researchers remain committed to discovering more peptide-based lead candidates and understanding their molecular mechanisms. For instance, Sifuvirtide has already entered clinical trials in China [87]. The development of these inhibitors holds promise for addressing the ongoing threat posed by viruses, including those that have the potential to cause pandemics. By continuing to explore and refine peptide-based fusion inhibitors, researchers aim to create more effective and broadly applicable antiviral drugs that can protect public health and respond to emerging viral threats.

Acknowledgements

We thank the financial support from the Inner Mongolia Natural Science Foundation of China (No. 2023LHMS08045;2025QN08006), the ZHIXUE Talent Project of Inner Mongolia Medical University 2024–2026 (No. ZY20241203), the Laboratory Open Fund Project of Inner Mongolia Medical University (No. 2024GZ17;2024ZN26), the Sub-project of Quality Enhancement and Cultivation Discipline for the Pharmacy College of Inner Mongolia Medical University (No. YXY2024TZ701), and Basic Research and Applied Basic Research Projects in Hohhot (No. 2024-规-基-20).

Author details

Guodong Liang[1,2]*, Yan Huang[1], Jinlin Wang[1], Xin Gao[1], Yuting Zhao[1], Lu Ga[1], Yan Zhao[1], Yuheng Ma[1], Yunfeng Xiao[1], Taoran Wang[3], Yihui Jin[1] and Ruijuan Li[1]

1 Key Laboratory for Candidate Drug Design and Screening Based on Chemical Biology, College of Pharmacy, Inner Mongolia Medical University, Hohhot, China

2 Zhen-Xiang Technology Co., Ltd, Hohhot, China

3 Beijing Institute of Pharmacology and Toxicology, Beijing, China

*Address all correspondence to: lgd08502214@163.com

References

[1] Seley-Radtke KL, Thames JE, Waters CD, 3rd. Broad spectrum antiviral nucleosides-our best hope for the future. Annual Reports in Medicinal Chemistry. 2021;**57**:109-132. DOI: 10.1016/bs.armc.2021.09.001

[2] Pattnaik GP, Chakraborty H. Entry inhibitors: Efficient means to block viral infection. The Journal of Membrane Biology. 2020;**253**(5):425-444. DOI: 10.1007/s00232-020-00136-z

[3] Vigant F, Santos NC, Lee B. Broad-spectrum antivirals against viral fusion. Nature Reviews. Microbiology. 2015;**13**(7):426-437. DOI: 10.1038/nrmicro3475

[4] Dimitrov DS. Virus entry: Molecular mechanisms and biomedical applications. Nature Reviews. Microbiology. 2004;**2**(2):109-122. DOI: 10.1038/nrmicro817

[5] Harrison SC. Mechanism of membrane fusion by viral envelope proteins. Advances in Virus Research. 2005;**64**:231-261. DOI: 10.1016/S0065-3527(05)64007-9

[6] Wyatt R, Sodroski J. The HIV-1 envelope glycoproteins: Fusogens, antigens, and immunogens. Science. 1998;**280**(5371):1884-1888. DOI: 10.1126/science.280.5371.1884

[7] Duzgunes N, Fernandez-Fuentes N, Konopka K. Inhibition of viral membrane fusion by peptides and approaches to peptide design. Pathogens. 2021;**10**(12):1599. DOI: 10.3390/pathogens10121599

[8] Schutz D, Ruiz-Blanco YB, Munch J, Kirchhoff F, Sanchez-Garcia E, Muller JA. Peptide and peptide-based inhibitors of SARS-CoV-2 entry. Advanced Drug Delivery Reviews. 2020;**167**:47-65. DOI: 10.1016/j.addr.2020.11.007

[9] Jiang S, Zhang X, Du L. Therapeutic antibodies and fusion inhibitors targeting the spike protein of SARS-CoV-2. Expert Opinion on Therapeutic Targets. 2021;**25**(6):415-421. DOI: 10.1080/14728222.2020.1820482

[10] Xiao T, Cai Y, Chen B. HIV-1 entry and membrane fusion inhibitors. Viruses. 2021;**13**(5):735. DOI: 10.3390/v13050735

[11] Moore JP, Doms RW. The entry of entry inhibitors: A fusion of science and medicine. Proceedings of the National Academy of Sciences of the United States of America. 2003;**100**(19):10598-10602. DOI: 10.1073/pnas.1932511100

[12] Eckert DM, Kim PS. Design of potent inhibitors of HIV-1 entry from the gp41 N-peptide region. Proceedings of the National Academy of Sciences of the United States of America. 2001;**98**(20):11187-11192. DOI: 10.1073/pnas.201392898

[13] Yi HA, Fochtman BC, Rizzo RC, Jacobs A. Inhibition of HIV entry by targeting the envelope transmembrane subunit gp41. Current HIV Research. 2016;**14**(3):283-294. DOI: 10.2174/1570162x14999160224103908

[14] Jiang S, Zhao Q, Debnath AK. Peptide and non-peptide HIV fusion inhibitors. Current Pharmaceutical Design. 2002;**8**(8):563-580. DOI: 10.2174/1381612024607180

[15] Binley JM, Wrin T, Korber B, Zwick MB, Wang M, Chappey C,

et al. Comprehensive cross-clade neutralization analysis of a panel of anti-human immunodeficiency virus type 1 monoclonal antibodies. Journal of Virology. 2004;**78**(23):13232-13252. DOI: 10.1128/JVI.78.23.13232-13252.2004

[16] Mascola JR, Lewis MG, Stiegler G, Harris D, Van Cott TC, Hayes D, et al. Protection of macaques against pathogenic simian/human immunodeficiency virus 89.6PD by passive transfer of neutralizing antibodies. Journal of Virology. 1999;**73**(5):4009-4018. DOI: 10.1128/JVI.73.5.4009-4018.1999

[17] Cai L, Jiang S. Development of peptide and small-molecule HIV-1 fusion inhibitors that target gp41. ChemMedChem. 2010;**5**(11):1813-1824. DOI: 10.1002/cmdc.201000289

[18] Zhang D, Li W, Jiang S. Peptide fusion inhibitors targeting the HIV-1 gp41: A patent review (2009-2014). Expert Opinion on Therapeutic Patents. 2015;**25**(2):159-173. DOI: 10.1517/13543776.2014.987752

[19] Chan DC, Chutkowski CT, Kim PS. Evidence that a prominent cavity in the coiled coil of HIV type 1 gp41 is an attractive drug target. Proceedings of the National Academy of Sciences of the United States of America. 1998;**95**(26):15613-15617. DOI: 10.1073/pnas.95.26.15613

[20] Chong H, Yao X, Qiu Z, Sun J, Zhang M, Waltersperger S, et al. Short-peptide fusion inhibitors with high potency against wild-type and enfuvirtide-resistant HIV-1. The FASEB Journal. 2013;**27**(3):1203-1213. DOI: 10.1096/fj.12-222547

[21] Otaka A, Nakamura M, Nameki D, Kodama E, Uchiyama S, Nakamura S, et al. Remodeling of gp41-C34 peptide leads to highly effective inhibitors of the fusion of HIV-1 with target cells. Angewandte Chemie (International Ed. in English). 2002;**41**(16):2937-2940. DOI: 10.1002/1521-3773(20020816)41:16<2937::AID-ANIE2937>3.0.CO;2-J

[22] Nishikawa H, Nakamura S, Kodama E, Ito S, Kajiwara K, Izumi K, et al. Electrostatically constrained alpha-helical peptide inhibits replication of HIV-1 resistant to enfuvirtide. The International Journal of Biochemistry & Cell Biology. 2009;**41**(4):891-899. DOI: 10.1016/j.biocel.2008.08.039

[23] Naito T, Izumi K, Kodama E, Sakagami Y, Kajiwara K, Nishikawa H, et al. SC29EK, a peptide fusion inhibitor with enhanced alpha-helicity, inhibits replication of human immunodeficiency virus type 1 mutants resistant to enfuvirtide. Antimicrobial Agents and Chemotherapy. 2009;**53**(3):1013-1018. DOI: 10.1128/AAC.01211-08

[24] Nishikawa H, Oishi S, Fujita M, Watanabe K, Tokiwa R, Ohno H, et al. Identification of minimal sequence for HIV-1 fusion inhibitors. Bioorganic & Medicinal Chemistry. 2008;**16**(20):9184-9187. DOI: 10.1016/j.bmc.2008.09.018

[25] Marqusee S, Baldwin RL. Helix stabilization by Glu-...Lys+ salt bridges in short peptides of de novo design. Proceedings of the National Academy of Sciences of the United States of America. 1987;**84**(24):8898-8902. DOI: 10.1073/pnas.84.24.8898

[26] McNaughton BR, Cronican JJ, Thompson DB, Liu DR. Mammalian cell penetration, siRNA transfection, and DNA transfection by supercharged proteins. Proceedings of the National Academy of Sciences of the United States of America. 2009;**106**(15):6111-6116. DOI: 10.1073/pnas.0807883106

[27] Cronican JJ, Thompson DB, Beier KT, McNaughton BR, Cepko CL, Liu DR. Potent delivery of functional proteins into mammalian cells in vitro and in vivo using a supercharged protein. ACS Chemical Biology. 2010;**5**(8):747-752. DOI: 10.1021/cb1001153

[28] Lawrence MS, Phillips KJ, Liu DR. Supercharging proteins can impart unusual resilience. Journal of the American Chemical Society. 2007;**129**(33):10110-10112. DOI: 10.1021/ja071641y

[29] Apostolopoulos V, Bojarska J, Chai TT, Elnagdy S, Kaczmarek K, Matsoukas J, et al. A global review on short peptides: Frontiers and perspectives. Molecules. 2021;**26**(2):430. DOI: 10.3390/molecules26020430

[30] Verdine GL, Walensky LD. The challenge of drugging undruggable targets in cancer: Lessons learned from targeting BCL-2 family members. Clinical Cancer Research. 2007;**13**(24):7264-7270. DOI: 10.1158/1078-0432.CCR-07-2184

[31] Bird GH, Madani N, Perry AF, Princiotto AM, Supko JG, He X, et al. Hydrocarbon double-stapling remedies the proteolytic instability of a lengthy peptide therapeutic. Proceedings of the National Academy of Sciences of the United States of America. 2010;**107**(32):14093-14098. DOI: 10.1073/pnas.1002713107

[32] Meng G, Pu J, Li Y, Han A, Tian Y, Xu W, et al. Design and biological evaluation of m-xylene thioether-stapled short helical peptides targeting the HIV-1 gp41 hexameric coiled-coil fusion complex. Journal of Medicinal Chemistry. 2019;**62**(19):8773-8783. DOI: 10.1021/acs.jmedchem.9b00882

[33] Wang C, Xia S, Zhang P, Zhang T, Wang W, Tian Y, et al. Discovery of hydrocarbon-stapled short alpha-helical peptides as promising middle east respiratory syndrome coronavirus (MERS-CoV) fusion inhibitors. Journal of Medicinal Chemistry. 2018;**61**(5):2018-2026. DOI: 10.1021/acs.jmedchem.7b01732

[34] Chong H, Yao X, Qiu Z, Qin B, Han R, Waltersperger S, et al. Discovery of critical residues for viral entry and inhibition through structural insight of HIV-1 fusion inhibitor CP621-652. The Journal of Biological Chemistry. 2012;**287**(24):20281-20289. DOI: 10.1074/jbc.M112.354126

[35] Yao X, Chong H, Zhang C, Qiu Z, Qin B, Han R, et al. Structural basis of potent and broad HIV-1 fusion inhibitor CP32M. The Journal of Biological Chemistry. 2012;**287**(32):26618-26629. DOI: 10.1074/jbc.M112.381079

[36] He Y, Cheng J, Lu H, Li J, Hu J, Qi Z, et al. Potent HIV fusion inhibitors against enfuvirtide-resistant HIV-1 strains. Proceedings of the National Academy of Sciences of the United States of America. 2008;**105**(42):16332-16337. DOI: 10.1073/pnas.0807335105

[37] Chong H, Yao X, Qiu Z, Sun J, Qiao Y, Zhang M, et al. The M-T hook structure increases the potency of HIV-1 fusion inhibitor sifuvirtide and overcomes drug resistance. The Journal of Antimicrobial Chemotherapy. 2014;**69**(10):2759-2769. DOI: 10.1093/jac/dku183

[38] Chong H, Qiu Z, Sun J, Qiao Y, Li X, He Y. Two M-T hook residues greatly improve the antiviral activity and resistance profile of the HIV-1 fusion inhibitor SC29EK. Retrovirology. 2014;**11**:40. DOI: 10.1186/1742-4690-11-40

[39] Liang G, Wang H, Chong H, Cheng S, Jiang X, He Y, et al. An effective

conjugation strategy for designing short peptide-based HIV-1 fusion inhibitors. Organic & Biomolecular Chemistry. 2016;**14**(33):7875-7882. DOI: 10.1039/c6ob01334a

[40] Weissenhorn W, Dessen A, Harrison SC, Skehel JJ, Wiley DC. Atomic structure of the ectodomain from HIV-1 gp41. Nature. 1997;**387**(6631):426-430. DOI: 10.1038/387426a0

[41] Zhu Y, Su S, Qin L, Wang Q, Shi L, Ma Z, et al. Rational improvement of gp41-targeting HIV-1 fusion inhibitors: An innovatively designed Ile-Asp-Leu tail with alternative conformations. Scientific Reports. 2016;**6**:31983. DOI: 10.1038/srep31983

[42] Su Y, Chong H, Qiu Z, Xiong S, He Y. Mechanism of HIV-1 resistance to short-peptide fusion inhibitors targeting the Gp41 pocket. Journal of Virology. 2015;**89**(11):5801-5811. DOI: 10.1128/JVI.00373-15

[43] Su S, Ma Z, Hua C, Li W, Lu L, Jiang S. Adding an artificial tail-anchor to a peptide-based HIV-1 fusion inhibitor for improvement of its potency and resistance profile. Molecules. 2017;**22**(11):1996. DOI: 10.3390/molecules22111996

[44] Su S, Zhu Y, Ye S, Qi Q, Xia S, Ma Z, et al. Creating an artificial tail anchor as a novel strategy to enhance the potency of peptide-based HIV fusion inhibitors. Journal of Virology. 2017;**91**(1):e01445-16. DOI: 10.1128/JVI.01445-16

[45] Su S, Rasquinha G, Du L, Wang Q, Xu W, Li W, et al. A peptide-based HIV-1 fusion inhibitor with two tail-anchors and palmitic acid exhibits substantially improved in vitro and ex vivo anti-HIV-1 activity and prolonged In vivo half-life. Molecules. 2019;**24**(6):1134. DOI: 10.3390/molecules24061134

[46] Fosgerau K, Hoffmann T. Peptide therapeutics: Current status and future directions. Drug Discovery Today. 2015;**20**(1):122-128. DOI: 10.1016/j.drudis.2014.10.003

[47] Otvos L Jr, Wade JD. Current challenges in peptide-based drug discovery. Frontiers in Chemistry. 2014;**2**:62. DOI: 10.3389/fchem.2014.00062

[48] Ferrer M, Kapoor TM, Strassmaier T, Weissenhorn W, Skehel JJ, Oprian D, et al. Selection of gp41-mediated HIV-1 cell entry inhibitors from biased combinatorial libraries of non-natural binding elements. Nature Structural Biology. 1999;**6**(10):953-960. DOI: 10.1038/13324

[49] Wang C, Shi W, Cai L, Lu L, Wang Q, Zhang T, et al. Design, synthesis, and biological evaluation of highly potent small molecule-peptide conjugates as new HIV-1 fusion inhibitors. Journal of Medicinal Chemistry. 2013;**56**(6):2527-2539. DOI: 10.1021/jm3018964

[50] Yu D, Sakurai Y, Chen CH, Chang FR, Huang L, Kashiwada Y, et al. Anti-AIDS agents 69. Moronic acid and other triterpene derivatives as novel potent anti-HIV agents. Journal of Medicinal Chemistry. 2006;**49**(18):5462-5469. DOI: 10.1021/jm0601912

[51] Mathieu C, Porotto M, Figueira TN, Horvat B, Moscona A. Fusion inhibitory lipopeptides engineered for prophylaxis of Nipah virus in primates. The Journal of Infectious Diseases. 2018;**218**(2):218-227. DOI: 10.1093/infdis/jiy152

[52] Simons K, Ikonen E. Functional rafts in cell membranes. Nature. 1997;**387**(6633):569-572. DOI: 10.1038/42408

[53] Viard M, Parolini I, Sargiacomo M, Fecchi K, Ramoni C, Ablan S,

et al. Role of cholesterol in human immunodeficiency virus type 1 envelope protein-mediated fusion with host cells. Journal of Virology. 2002;**76**(22):11584-11595. DOI: 10.1128/jvi.76.22.11584-11595.2002

[54] Nguyen DH, Hildreth JE. Evidence for budding of human immunodeficiency virus type 1 selectively from glycolipid-enriched membrane lipid rafts. Journal of Virology. 2000;**74**(7):3264-3272. DOI: 10.1128/jvi.74.7.3264-3272.2000

[55] Ono A, Freed EO. Plasma membrane rafts play a critical role in HIV-1 assembly and release. Proceedings of the National Academy of Sciences of the United States of America. 2001;**98**(24):13925-13930. DOI: 10.1073/pnas.241320298

[56] Wexler-Cohen Y, Shai Y. Demonstrating the C-terminal boundary of the HIV 1 fusion conformation in a dynamic ongoing fusion process and implication for fusion inhibition. The FASEB Journal. 2007;**21**(13):3677-3684. DOI: 10.1096/fj.07-8582com

[57] Ingallinella P, Bianchi E, Ladwa NA, Wang YJ, Hrin R, Veneziano M, et al. Addition of a cholesterol group to an HIV-1 peptide fusion inhibitor dramatically increases its antiviral potency. Proceedings of the National Academy of Sciences of the United States of America. 2009;**106**(14):5801-5806. DOI: 10.1073/pnas.0901007106

[58] Hollmann A, Matos PM, Augusto MT, Castanho MA, Santos NC. Conjugation of cholesterol to HIV-1 fusion inhibitor C34 increases peptide-membrane interactions potentiating its action. PLoS One. 2013;**8**(4):e60302. DOI: 10.1371/journal.pone.0060302

[59] Ashkenazi A, Viard M, Unger L, Blumenthal R, Shai Y. Sphingopeptides: Dihydrosphingosine-based fusion inhibitors against wild-type and enfuvirtide-resistant HIV-1. The FASEB Journal. 2012;**26**(11):4628-4636. DOI: 10.1096/fj.12-215111

[60] Wexler-Cohen Y, Ashkenazi A, Viard M, Blumenthal R, Shai Y. Virus-cell and cell-cell fusion mediated by the HIV-1 envelope glycoprotein is inhibited by short gp41 N-terminal membrane-anchored peptides lacking the critical pocket domain. The FASEB Journal. 2010;**24**(11):4196-4202. DOI: 10.1096/fj.09-151704

[61] Augusto MT, Hollmann A, Castanho MA, Porotto M, Pessi A, Santos NC. Improvement of HIV fusion inhibitor C34 efficacy by membrane anchoring and enhanced exposure. The Journal of Antimicrobial Chemotherapy. 2014;**69**(5):1286-1297. DOI: 10.1093/jac/dkt529

[62] Chong H, Xue J, Xiong S, Cong Z, Ding X, Zhu Y, et al. A lipopeptide HIV-1/2 fusion inhibitor with highly potent in vitro, ex vivo, and in vivo antiviral activity. Journal of Virology. 2017;**91**(11):e00288-17. DOI: 10.1128/JVI.00288-17

[63] Wang H, Wang C. Peptide-based dual HIV and coronavirus entry inhibitors. Advances in Experimental Medicine and Biology. 2022;**1366**:87-100. DOI: 10.1007/978-981-16-8702-0_6

[64] Na H, Luo H, Wang J, Sun L, Gao X, Liang G, et al. An N-terminal heptad repeat trimer-based peptide fusion inhibitor exhibits potent anti-H1N1 activity. Bioorganic & Medicinal Chemistry. 2024;**111**:117865. DOI: 10.1016/j.bmc.2024.117865

[65] Clinton TR, Weinstock MT, Jacobsen MT, Szabo-Fresnais N, Pandya MJ, Whitby FG, et al. Design and characterization of ebolavirus GP

prehairpin intermediate mimics as drug targets. Protein Science. 2015;**24**(4):446-463. DOI: 10.1002/pro.2578

[66] Matthews JM, Young TF, Tucker SP, Mackay JP. The core of the respiratory syncytial virus fusion protein is a trimeric coiled coil. Journal of Virology. 2000;**74**(13):5911-5920. DOI: 10.1128/jvi.74.13.5911-5920.2000

[67] Wang J, Li P, Li R, Liang G, Ma Y, Na H. Structural basis of HIV-1 gp41 N-trimer for designing bifunctional peptide-based fusion inhibitors. Current Medicinal Chemistry. 2025;**32**(25):5321-5337. DOI: 10.2174/010929867 3291459240328074404

[68] Bewley CA, Louis JM, Ghirlando R, Clore GM. Design of a novel peptide inhibitor of HIV fusion that disrupts the internal trimeric coiled-coil of gp41. The Journal of Biological Chemistry. 2002;**277**(16):14238-14245. DOI: 10.1074/jbc.M201453200

[69] Kang HJ, Coulibaly F, Clow F, Proft T, Baker EN. Stabilizing isopeptide bonds revealed in gram-positive bacterial pilus structure. Science. 2007;**318**(5856):1625-1628. DOI: 10.1126/science.1145806

[70] Zakeri B, Fierer JO, Celik E, Chittock EC, Schwarz-Linek U, Moy VT, et al. Peptide tag forming a rapid covalent bond to a protein, through engineering a bacterial adhesin. Proceedings of the National Academy of Sciences of the United States of America. 2012;**109**(12):E690-E697. DOI: 10.1073/pnas.1115485109

[71] Fierer JO, Veggiani G, Howarth M. SpyLigase peptide-peptide ligation polymerizes affibodies to enhance magnetic cancer cell capture. Proceedings of the National Academy of Sciences of the United States of America. 2014;**111**(13):E1176-E1181. DOI: 10.1073/pnas.1315776111

[72] Brune KD, Leneghan DB, Brian IJ, Ishizuka AS, Bachmann MF, Draper SJ, et al. Plug-and-display: Decoration of virus-like particles via isopeptide bonds for modular immunization. Scientific Reports. 2016;**6**:19234. DOI: 10.1038/srep19234

[73] Zakeri B, Howarth M. Spontaneous intermolecular amide bond formation between side chains for irreversible peptide targeting. Journal of the American Chemical Society. 2010;**132**(13):4526-4527. DOI: 10.1021/ja910795a

[74] Wang C, Lai W, Yu F, Zhang T, Lu L, Jiang X, et al. De novo design of isopeptide bond-tethered triple-stranded coiled coils with exceptional resistance to unfolding and proteolysis: Implication for developing antiviral therapeutics. Chemical Science. 2015;**6**(11):6505-6509. DOI: 10.1039/c5sc02220g

[75] Fletcher JM, Boyle AL, Bruning M, Bartlett GJ, Vincent TL, Zaccai NR, et al. A basis set of de novo coiled-coil peptide oligomers for rational protein design and synthetic biology. ACS Synthetic Biology. 2012;**1**(6):240-250. DOI: 10.1021/sb300028q

[76] Bai Y, Xue H, Ling Y, Cheng M, Cai L, Liu K. Inter-chain acyl transfer reaction in a peptide six-helical bundle: A chemical method for regulating the interaction between peptides or proteins. Chemical Communications (Camb). 2012;**48**(36):4320-4322. DOI: 10.1039/c2cc17428f

[77] Bai Y, Wang C, Liang G, Lai W, Xue H, Ling Y, et al. Precisely designed isopeptide bridge-crosslinking endows artificial hydrolases with high stability and catalytic activity under extreme

denaturing conditions. Chemistry, an Asian Journal. 2017;**12**(19):2539-2543. DOI: 10.1002/asia.201701021

[78] Lai W, Wang C, Yan J, Liu H, Zhang W, Lin B, et al. Suitable fusion of N-terminal heptad repeats to achieve covalently stabilized potent N-peptide inhibitors of HIV-1 infection. Bioorganic & Medicinal Chemistry. 2020;**28**(4):115214. DOI: 10.1016/j.bmc.2019.115214

[79] Chan DC, Fass D, Berger JM, Kim PS. Core structure of gp41 from the HIV envelope glycoprotein. Cell. 1997;**89**(2):263-273. DOI: 10.1016/s0092-8674(00)80205-6

[80] Lai W, Wang C, Yu F, Lu L, Wang Q, Jiang X, et al. An effective strategy for recapitulating N-terminal heptad repeat trimers in enveloped virus surface glycoproteins for therapeutic applications. Chemical Science. 2016;**7**(3):2145-2150. DOI: 10.1039/c5sc04046a

[81] Huang Y, Luo H, Jin Y, Ma Y, Zhao Y, Gao X, et al. Design of coiled-coil N-peptides against HIV-1 based on a CADD strategy. Organic & Biomolecular Chemistry. 2024;**23**(1):157-166. DOI: 10.1039/d4ob01620c

[82] Wang C, Xia S, Wang X, Li Y, Wang H, Xiang R, et al. Supercoiling structure-based design of a trimeric coiled-coil peptide with high potency against HIV-1 and human beta-coronavirus infection. Journal of Medicinal Chemistry. 2022;**65**(4):2809-2819. DOI: 10.1021/acs.jmedchem.1c00258

[83] Heydari H, Golmohammadi R, Mirnejad R, Tebyanian H, Fasihi-Ramandi M, Moosazadeh Moghaddam M. Antiviral peptides against coronaviridae family: A review. Peptides. 2021;**139**:170526. DOI: 10.1016/j.peptides.2021.170526

[84] Bode SA, Kruis IC, Adams HP, Boelens WC, Pruijn GJ, van Hest JC, et al. Coiled-coil-mediated activation of oligoarginine cell-penetrating peptides. Chembiochem. 2017;**18**(2):185-188. DOI: 10.1002/cbic.201600614

[85] Gump JM, Dowdy SF. TAT transduction: The molecular mechanism and therapeutic prospects. Trends in Molecular Medicine. 2007;**13**(10):443-448. DOI: 10.1016/j.molmed.2007.08.002

[86] Pu J, Wang Q, Jiang S. Peptide-based HIV entry inhibitors. Advances in Experimental Medicine and Biology. 2022;**1366**:15-26. DOI: 10.1007/978-981-16-8702-0_2

[87] Yu D, Ding X, Liu Z, Wu X, Zhu Y, Wei H, et al. Molecular mechanism of HIV-1 resistance to sifuvirtide, a clinical trial-approved membrane fusion inhibitor. The Journal of Biological Chemistry. 2018;**293**(33):12703-12718. DOI: 10.1074/jbc.RA118.003538

Section 4

Clinical Challenges in Viral Respiratory Diseases

Chapter 5

Investigation of the Frequency of Atypical Pneumonia and Viral Pneumonia in Pneumonia Cases in Intensive Care Units

Ahmet Doğan, Yasemin Ersoy Çinar, Bariş Otlu and Çiğdem Kuzucu

Abstract

Many causative pathogens can cause pneumonia. Atypical pathogens such as *Legionella pneumophila, Mycoplasma pneumoniae, Chlamydophila pneumoniae* and *Chlamydia psittaci* are important known agents of atypical pneumonia. Viruses can cause pneumonia in both immunocompetent and immunocompromised patients. As causative pathogens, Adenovirus (AV), Meta-pneumovirus (MPV), Para-influenza virus (PIV), Respiratory syncytial virus (RSV) and Influenza A (Inf A) and B (Inf B) virus usually have mild clinical manifestations and a good prognosis. However, Herpes Virus (HSV), Cytomegalovirus (CMV) and Epstein-Barr Virus (EBV) have high mortality in immunosuppressives In this prospective, cross-sectional, single center study, we aimed to determine the causative agents of atypical pneumonia and viral pneumonia in cases requiring intensive care unit due to pneumonia. The prognosis of the cases was also analyzed.

Keywords: viral pneumoniae, intensive care unit, community-acquired pneumoniae, hospital-acquired pneumoniae, atypical pneumonia

1. Introduction

Many causative pathogens can cause pneumonia. Atypical pathogens such as *Legionella pneumophila, Mycoplasma pneumoniae, Chlamydophila pneumoniae,* and *Chlamydia psittaci* are important known agents of atypical pneumonia. It may not always be clinically possible to distinguish between typical and atypical pneumonia pathogens [1]. Rapid diagnosis and treatment are important to reduce mortality and septic shock [2]. Urine antigen testing and molecular tests (PCR) have high sensitivity, especially in the diagnosis of atypical agents [3]. *L. pneumoniae* varies according to geographical locations, but generally, one-fifth of cases require intensive care [4]. *M. pneumoniae* can cause upper and lower respiratory tract infections. It can have a

30% mortality rate, especially in the geriatric age group [5, 6]. Similar to other atypical agents, *C. pneumoniae* may present with different clinical severity [7]. Viruses can cause pneumonia in both immunocompetent and immunocompromised patients. Especially in immunosuppressed patients, the frequency is increasing day by day. Clinical presentation in adults is very variable. It can range from mild clinical manifestations to severe pneumonia shock and mechanical ventilation. It can be seen as a causative agent in both community-acquired (CAP) and hospital-acquired pneumonias (HAP) [8]. As causative pathogens, *Adenovirus (AV), Meta-pneumovirus (MPV), Para-influenza virus (PIV), Respiratory syncytial virus (RSV),* and *Influenza A (Inf A)* and *B (Inf B)* virus usually have mild clinical manifestations and a good prognosis. However, *Herpes Virus (HSV), Cytomegalovirus (CMV),* and *Epstein-Barr Virus (EBV)* have high mortality in immunosuppressives [9]. In this prospective, cross-sectional, single-center study, we aimed to determine the causative agents of atypical pneumonia and viral pneumonia in cases requiring intensive care unit due to pneumonia. The prognosis of the cases was also analyzed.

2. Materials and methods

The study was planned between November 1, 2016 and October 30, 2017. A total of 200 pneumonia cases were included. Cases aged 18 years and older, CAP and HAP cases were included. Patients under 18 years of age, patients with hematologic malignancies, organ transplant patients, neutropenic patients, and patients with HIV diagnosis were excluded. In addition, patients with a diagnosis of pneumonia whose antibacterial treatment duration was more than 72 hours were excluded from the study.

3. Parameters

The complaints, radiologic findings, history of antibiotic usage, demographic data, and laboratory values of the patients to be followed up in the study were recorded. APACHE II score of each patient was also calculated. Tracheal aspirate and sputum culture, virus PCR and Legionella BCYE culture results, antibacterial treatments, and prognosis of the patients were recorded.

4. Diagnosis of pneumonia

The diagnosis of pneumonia was based on the Turkish Thoracic Society Consensus Report on the Diagnosis and Treatment of Community-Acquired Pneumonia in Adults 2009 and Infectious Diseases Society of America/American Thoracic Society Consensus Guidelines on the Management of Community-Acquired Pneumonia in Adults 2007 [10, 11].

5. Microbiological and molecular methods

Tracheal aspirate and sputum cultures were performed for the detection of atypical pneumonia pathogens *M. pneumoniae, C. pneumoniae*, and *L. pneumophiliae*. In addition, BCYE culture was performed in the same samples for the detection of *L.*

pneumophiliae. For the isolation of *RSV, human metapneumovirus (HMPV), rhinovirus (RV), enterovirus (EV), parainfluenza virus (PIV), Inf A, Inf B, human bocavirus (HBoV), adenovirus*, specific DNA/RNA was investigated by in-house multiplex PCR method from nasopharynx swab samples.

6. Study design

For the study, DNA/RNA extraction kit for bacterial and viral DNA/RNA isolation, SYBR Green PCR kit and Primer Standard for PCR, BCYE Growth Supplement without L-cysteine, BCYE Growth Supplement with L-cysteine addition, Legionella GVPC Supplement with antibiotic addition, and BCYE Legionella supplements were prepared in the laboratory with the coordination support of scientific research projects (BAP) number 39/2016. After demonstrating that the nutrient and multiplex PCR method worked with positive controls, the patient form was created.

7. Ethics committee approval

For the approval of the study, the "Clinical Research Ethics Committee Decision Form" was created on June 08, 2016. According to this form, the necessary permission was received for the study with protocol number 2016/116.

8. Statistical analysis

Data was entered into the IBM SPSS Statistics 22 package program for analysis. Continuous and discrete quantitative variables in the data were summarized as median (min-max) and qualitative variables as number (percentage). Kolmogorov Smirnov and Shapiro-Wilk tests were used to determine whether the data were normally distributed. The Mann-Whitney U test was used to analyze statistically significant differences between group variable categories in terms of continuous and intermittent quantitative variables. Pearson's chi-square, Yates corrected chi-square, and Fisher's exact chi-square tests were used to determine the significance between categorical data. $p < 0.05$ was accepted as the level of statistical significance.

9. Results

A total of 200 pneumonia cases from five intensive care units were included in the study. Of the patients, 126 (63%) were male and 74 (37%) were female. The mean age of all patients was 62.8 ± 18.09 years. 65 (32.5%) of the patients were CAP and 135 (67.5%) were HAP. The majority of cases belonged to the Reanimation ICU (**Figure 1**).

Fever was observed in 32.5% of patients, dyspnea in 61%, tachypnea in 56%, purulent sputum in 95.5%, and increased cough in 7.5%. Symptoms of the patients according to source are summarized in **Table 1**.

All patients had areas of infiltration on lung radiography. 65 (32.5%) patients were extubated and 135 (67.5%) were intubated. Twenty-three (20%) patients had PaO2/FiO2 of 400 or more, 28 (14%) patients had 399–300, 74 (37%) patients had 299–150, and 58 (29%) patients had <150. In the laboratory values of the patients,

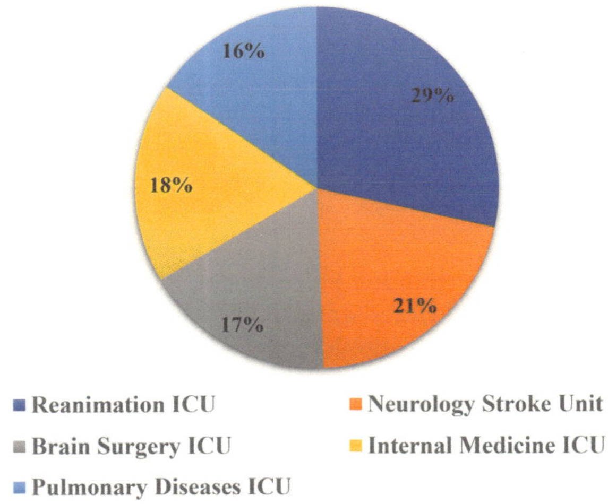

Figure 1.
Intensive care units included in the study and patient percentages.

The variables	CAP	HAP	*p*-value
Gender			
• Male	50 (76.9)	76 (56.2)	**<0.008**
• Female	15 (23.1)	59 (43.8)	
Age (mean ± SD)	(65.68 ± 16.9)	(61.42 ± 18.53)	>0.05
Origin	65 (32.5)	135 (57.5)	—
Symptom			
• Fire	19 (29.2)	46 (34)	>0.05
• Dyspnea	39 (60)	83 (61.4)	>0.05
• Takipne	33 (50.7)	79 (58.5)	>0.05
• Purulent sputum	61 (93.8)	130 (96.2)	>0.05
• Increased cough	3 (4.6)	12 (8.8)	>0.05

Table 1.
Demographic characteristics of the patients included in the study.

the white blood cell count was above the upper limit of the normal value in 159 (79.5%) patients. It was at or below the lower limit of normal value in four (2%) patients. There was a statistically significant difference between the source categories (community-acquired vs. hospital-acquired) in terms of white blood cell variables ($p < 0.049$). The CRP value studied in a total of 192 patients was above the normal limit in 189 (98.4%) patients. PCT was >0.5 in 55 (94.8%) of 58 patients. There was no statistically significant difference between CAP and HAP patient groups in terms of CRP and PCT variables ($p > 0.05$). History of quinolone or macrolide antibiotic usage in the last 3 days was present in 32 (16%) of the patients. APACHE II Score was calculated in all patients. There was no statistically significant difference in APACHE II Score between CAP and HAP patient groups ($p > 0.05$). In addition, no statistically significant difference was found between CAP and HAP patient groups in terms of PaO2/FiO2 ($p > 0.05$), (**Table 2**).

The variables	CAP (N = 65), (%)	HAP (N = 135), (%)	*p*-value
Antibiotic usage (last 3 days)			
• Quinolone or macrolide	16 (24.6)	16 (11.8)	*<0.036*
Consolidation on chest radiography	65 (100)	135 (100)	—
PaO2/FiO2			
• >400 • 399–300 • 299–150 • <150	9 (13.8) 9 (13.8) 29 (44.6) 18 (27.8)	20 (14.8) 20 (14.8) 45 (40.8) 40 (29.6)	>0.05
Ventilation			
• Extubated • Intubated	21 (32.3) 44 (67.7)	46 (34) 89 (66)	- -
APACHE II Score	17.38 ± 6.28	16.69 ± 5.53	>0.05
WBC			
• >10.000 • ≤4.500	47 (72.3) 1 (1.5)	99 (73.3) 3 (2.2)	*<0.049*
C-Reactive Protein			
• >0.5 • ≤0.5	- -	125 (92.5) 2 (1.5)	>0.05
Procalcitonin			
• >0.5 • ≤0.5	24 (94.8) -	31 (23) 3 (2.2)	>0.05
Prognosis			
• Excitus • Discharged	11 (17) 54 (83)	40 (29.6) 91 (70.4)	>0.05

Table 2.
Antibiotic use, radiology, APACHE II score, laboratory findings and intubation, mortality, PaO2/FiO2 ratios of patients.

Sub-diseases of all patients were recorded. In a total of 189 patients, other diseases were found to accompany pneumonia. Cerebrovascular accident, COPD, Trauma, Heart failure, coronary artery disease were the most common comorbidities (**Table 3**).

Tracheal aspirate culture (TAC) was performed in 82.5% and sputum culture in 17.5% of the patients. There was no growth in 89 of the patients with TAC. 76 patients grew typical pneumonia agents. Eight of the patients in whom sputum cultures were performed grew typical pneumonia agents. Of the 115 patients in whom no growth was detected in TAC and sputum culture, 28 patients died. When the pathogens detected by bacterial culture and PCR method were analyzed, no pathogen could be isolated in 39% of the cases. In most of the others, only bacterial pathogens, some viruses, and to a lesser extent, bacteria+viral pathogens and mycoplasma were detected (**Figure 2**).

Komorbidity	**CAP (N = 65), (%)**	**HAP (N = 135), (%)**
Cardiovascular Pathologies n = 52		
• Coronary artery disease	(7.5)	3 (1.8)
• Heart failure	(8.8)	11 (6.8)
• Atrial fibrillation	-	7 (4.3)
• Hypertension	5 (6.3)	6 (3.7)
• Cardiac arrest	4 (5)	3 (1.8)
Central Nervous System Pathologies n = 90		
• Cerebrovascular event	15 (19)	42 (26)
• Alzheimer's disease	7 (8.8)	6 (3.7)
• Cranial surgery	2 (2.5)	11 (6.8)
• Epileptic seizure	-	(1.8)
• Encephalitis	-	(2.5)
Malignancies n = 14	2 (2.5)	12 (7.4)
Pulmonary Pathologies n = 33		
• COPD	-	15 (9.3)
• Pulmonary edema	-	2 (1.2)
• Respiratory distress	-	1 (0.6)
Endocrine Pathologies n = 13		
• Diabetes mellitus	7 (8.8)	6 (3.7)
Renal Pathologies n = 13		
• Chronic renal failure	4 (5)	6 (3.7)
• Acute renal failure	3 (3.8)	-
Other n = 25		
• Trauma	1 (1.2)	19 (12)
• Abdominal surgery	-	3 (1.8)
• Drug intoxication	1 (1.2)	-
• Electric shock	-	1 (0.6)

CAP: Community Acquired Pneumonia, HAP: Hospital-acquired Pneumonia, COPD: Chronic Obstructive Pulmonary Disease.

Table 3.
Comorbid conditions of patients.

Cases were evaluated separately as CAP and HAP. Among typical CAP agents, the most common bacterial pathogen was K. pneumonia, while the most common viral pathogen was Rhinovirus and Influenza A. Among atypical pneumonia agents, only *M. pneumoniae* was detected. When HAP agents were analyzed, *Stapyhlococcus aureus* was the most common typical pneumonia agent, while Rhinovirus and Coronavirus were the most common viral agents. Among atypical agents, only *M. pneumoniae* was detected (**Figure 3**).

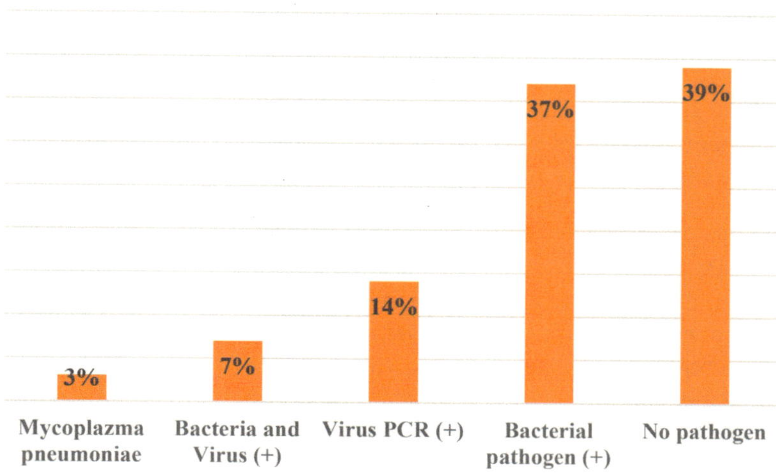

Figure 2.
The distribution of pathogens detected in cases.

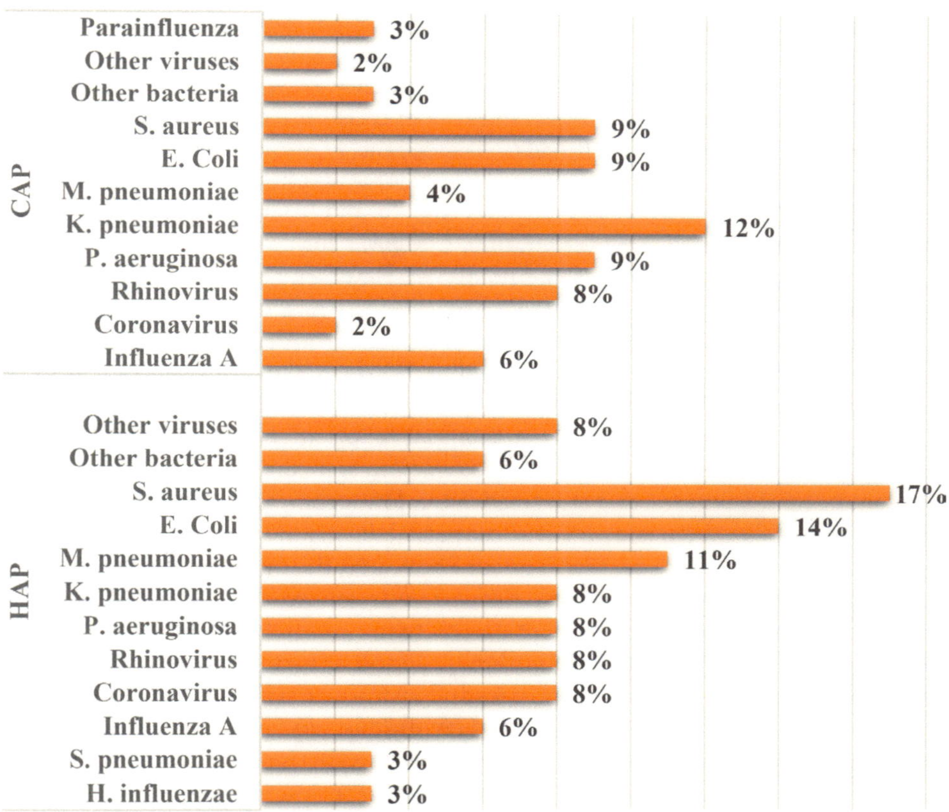

Figure 3.
Factors detected in community-acquired and hospital-acquired pneumonia cases ($p < 0.05$).

10. Discussion

In our country, routine culture or PCR is not performed in every center for the detection of atypical pneumonia agents in cases requiring intensive care due to HAP or CAP. When pneumonia treatment is planned, empirical treatment is usually planned to include atypical agents. Therefore, in this study, we investigated the rate of atypical and viral agents in intensive care unit cases at our center. Different rates are reported in foreign studies. In the Slovenian study, in SARS-CoV-2 cases, in 1472 lower respiratory tract samples, EBV, HSV-1, and CMV positivity rates were the most common with 74.7%, 58.1%, and 38.0%, respectively [10]. In another study of severe CAP cases, atypical pneumonia was detected in 26 patients among 856 patients. These included 18 *L. pneumophila* serogroup 1, 3 *M. pneumonia,* and 5 *C. psittaci*. Urine antigen was positive in 16 (89%) of Legionella cases. The diagnosis was also confirmed by PCR. However, there was no growth in culture [11]. In the Indian study, bacterial pathogens were detected in 266 (46.3%) of 574 CAPs. These were most commonly *K. pneumoniae* (33.6%) and *S. pneumoniae* (32.9%). Atypical pathogens (*Mycoplasma, Legionella,* and *Chlamydia*) were reported in 15.1% [12]. In a study of 311 cases in Turkey, the causative agent was isolated in 214 (68.8%) of the cases. 360 isolates were reported, including 338 viruses and 22 bacterial pathogens. The most common isolates were *influenza A + B* (18.1%), *hBoV* (17.8%), *RV/EV* (15.6%), and *RSV* (13.1%). Again, in different studies conducted in our country, *Influenza* and *Rhinovirus* virus came to the forefront [13–15]. Again, in another study examining the possibility that exacerbation may develop secondary to atypical pathogens in COPD patients in our country, culture positivity was 46%, while this rate increased to 85.1% when PCR was also performed. In 53.3% of cases, exacerbation was caused by multiple pathogens, of which 37.3% had two pathogens, 15% had three pathogens, and 0.9% had four pathogens. The presence of *H. influenzae* was shown in 58.9% of cases, *S. pneumoniae* in 53.2%, *Pseudomonas aeruginosa* in 14%, and *L. pneumophila* in 10.3% [16]. In our study, partially similar to the literature, *Legionella* cultures were not grown in any patient. Urine antigen for *Legionella* was not tested. However, no *Legionella* or *Chlamidia* was detected in PCR, while *Mycoplasma* was detected in 4% of cases. Considering these results, it can be concluded that *Legionella* or *Chlamidia* is not a significant problem in our pneumonia cases in the intensive care unit. However, the quality of respiratory specimens, missing BAL specimens, and deficiencies in the anamnesis of the relatives of intubated patients in our center are other potential factors affecting this result. Among the viral agents, *Rhinovirus, Coronavirus,* and *Influenza* were the most common agents. However, the reason why the rate of influenza was lower compared to other studies may be due to the fact that there was no pandemic period during the study period, as well as the inclusion of the summer period. In pneumonia cases, the frequency of typical agents such as *Acinetobacter*, *Pseudomonas,* and *Klepsiella* was noteworthy.

Pneumonia is an important cause of mortality in cases followed up in intensive care units. In addition, comorbid conditions are another factor that increases mortality [17–19]. In our study, 17% of CAP cases and 29.6% of HAP cases had a mortal prognosis. The presence of many comorbid conditions, especially central nervous system and cardiovascular diseases, was demonstrated in the cases.

The association of CRP and chest radiography in the diagnosis has been found to be significant especially in CAP [20]. In initial treatment, PCT study is not recommended. The presence of pulmonary symptoms at presentation, pneumonia severity scoring, and vital signs are valuable in the diagnosis [21–23]. When CAP and HAP were evaluated separately, gender emerged as an important factor in the development of pneumonia, while no significant difference was observed in terms of symptoms.

DOI: http://dx.doi.org/10.5772/intechopen.1005903

When laboratory values were analyzed, while CRP and PCT values were similar, leukocytosis was significantly higher in cases. Again, there was no significant difference in PaO2/FiO2, APACHE II score, intubation, and mortality. However, the history of quinolone or macrolide usage in the last 3 days was significantly higher in CAPs.

11. Conclusion

According to the results of our study, it was shown that atypical pneumonia agents were not in the first place in CAP and HAP in cases admitted to our center. It was observed that the cases generally presented with purulent sputum. The lower-than-expected incidence of fever may have been because the cases were generally from the older age group. *S. aureus* was most frequently isolated in HAP. Fortunately, Methicillin-resistant isolates are very rare in our center. This should be taken into consideration in empirical treatment. In HAPs, as expected, Gram-negative bacteria, especially *Acinetobacter*, were the most common causative agents. In addition to anamnesis, laboratory, and radiology, PCR significantly increases the detection rate of viral and atypical bacterial agents. *Rhinovirus* (8%) and *Coronavirus* (8%) were the most common viral agents detected in CAP patients, influenza was the third most common viral agent (6%). In HAPs, the most common viral agents were *Rhinovirus* (8%) and *Influenza* (6%). *Rhinovirus* and *Influenza* virus pneumonia should not be ignored, especially in the elderly patient group and patients in need of ICU. The high mortality rate in the group in which no causative agent was detected suggests that there may be undetected viral agents and atypical agents in this group and that mortality was high for this reason. Although atypical pneumonia and viral pneumonia do not seem to be an important problem in our center, there is a need for multicenter, prospective studies including a large number of cases in terms of national data.

Author details

Ahmet Doğan[1*], Yasemin Ersoy Çinar[2], Bariş Otlu[3] and Çiğdem Kuzucu[4]

1 Faculty of Medicine, Department of Infectious Diseases and Microbiology, Abant İzzet Baysal University, Bolu, Turkey

2 Faculty of Medicine, Department of Infectious Diseases and Microbiology, İnönü University, Malatya, Turkey

3 Faculty of Medicine, Department of Medical Microbiology, İnönü University, Malatya, Turkey

4 Faculty of Medicine, Department of Medical Microbiology, Tınaztepe University, İzmir, Turkey

*Address all correspondence to: uzdrahmetdogan@gmail.com

References

[1] Gacouin A, Revest M, Letheulle J, Fillatre P, Jouneau S, Piau C, et al. Distinctive features between community-acquired pneumonia (CAP) due to *Chlamydophila psittaci* and CAP due to *Legionella pneumophila* admitted to the intensive care unit (ICU). European Journal of Clinical Microbiology and Infectious Diseases: Official Publication of the European Society of Clinical Microbiology. 2012;**31**(10):2713-2718. DOI: 10.1007/s10096-012-1618-6

[2] Garnacho-Montero J, Garcia-Garmendia JL, Barrero-Almodovar A, Jimenez-Jimenez FJ, Perez-Paredes C, Ortiz-Leyba C. Impact of adequate empirical antibiotic therapy on the outcome of patients admitted to the intensive care unit with sepsis. Critical Care Medicine. 2003;**31**(12):2742-2751. DOI: 10.1097/01.CCM.0000098031.24329.10

[3] Cunha BA. The atypical pneumonias: Clinical diagnosis and importance. Clinical Microbiology and Infection: The Official Publication of the European Society of Clinical Microbiology and Infectious Diseases. 2006;**12**(Suppl. 3):12-24. DOI: 10.1111/j.1469-0691.2006.01393.x

[4] Falcone M, Russo A, Tiseo G, Cesaretti M, Guarracino F, Menichetti F. Predictors of intensive care unit admission in patients with *Legionella pneumonia*: Role of the time to appropriate antibiotic therapy. Infection. 2021;**49**(2):321-325. DOI: 10.1007/s15010-020-01565-7

[5] Lee H, Yun KW, Lee HJ, Choi EH. Antimicrobial therapy of macrolide-resistant *Mycoplasma pneumoniae* pneumonia in children. Expert Review of Anti-Infective Therapy. 2018;**16**(1):23-34. DOI: 10.1080/14787210.2018.1414599

[6] Hu J, Ye Y, Chen X, Xiong L, Xie W, Liu P. Insight into the pathogenic mechanism of *Mycoplasma pneumoniae*. Current Microbiology. 2022;**80**(1):14. DOI: 10.1007/s00284-022-03103-0

[7] Miyashita N. Atypical pneumonia: Pathophysiology, diagnosis, and treatment. Respiratory Investigation. 2022;**60**(1):56-67. DOI: 10.1016/j.resinv.2021.09.009

[8] Dandachi D, Rodriguez-Barradas MC. Viral pneumonia: Etiologies and treatment. Journal of Investigative Medicine: The Official Publication of the American Federation for Clinical Research. 2018;**66**(6):957-965. DOI: 10.1136/jim-2018-000712

[9] Almeida A, Boattini M, Christaki E, Moreira Marques T, Moreira I, Cruz L, et al. Comparative virulence of seasonal viruses responsible for lower respiratory tract infections: A southern European multi-centre cohort study of hospital admissions. Infection. 2021;**49**(3):483-490. DOI: 10.1007/s15010-020-01569-3

[10] Mandell LA, Wunderink RG, Anzueto A, Bartlett JG, Campbell GD, Dean NC, et al. Infectious Diseases Society of America/American Thoracic Society consensus guidelines on the management of community-acquired pneumonia in adults. Clinical Infectious Diseases: An Official Publication of the Infectious Diseases Society of America. 2007;**44**(Suppl. 2):S27-S72. DOI: 10.1086/511159

[11] Özlü T, Bülbül Y, Alataş F. Diagnosis and treatment consensus report for pneumonia developing in the community in adults. Turkish Thoracic Journal. 2009;**10**(Suppl. 9):1-18

[12] Grubelnik G, Korva M, Kogoj R, et al. Herpesviridae and atypical bacteria co-detections in lower respiratory tract samples of SARS-CoV-2-positive patients admitted to an intensive care unit. Microorganisms. 2024;**12**(4):714. Published 2024 Mar 31. DOI: 10.3390/microorganisms12040714

[13] Guillot P, Delamaire F, Gacouin A, Painvin B, Piau C, Reizine F, et al. Early discontinuation of combination antibiotic therapy in severe community-acquired pneumonia: A retrospective cohort study. BMC Infectious Diseases. 2023;**23**(1):611. DOI: 10.1186/s12879-023-08493-5

[14] Kalita D, Sarma RK, Sharma KR, Deka S. High proportion of drug-resistant isolates in adult community-acquired pneumonia from Northeast India: A hospital-based study. Lung India. 2021;**38**(5):460-465. DOI: 10.4103/lungindia.lungindia_978_20

[15] Harun A, Beyza E. Viral and atypical bacterial respiratory infections in a university teaching hospital. Japanese Journal of Infectious Diseases. 2019;**72**(5):318-322. DOI: 10.7883/yoken.JJID.2018.510

[16] Çörtük M, Acat M, Yazici O, Yasar Z, Kiraz K, Ataman SY, et al. Retrospective review of epidemic viral pneumonia cases in Turkey: A multicenter study. Experimental and Therapeutic Medicine. 2017;**13**(4):1431-1437. DOI: 10.3892/etm.2017.4153

[17] Ozlu T, Bülbül Y, Taşbakan S, Kılıç H, Kuyucu T, Yıldız T, et al. General characteristics and prognostic factors of pneumonia cases developed during pandemic (H1N1) influenza-a virus infection in Turkey. Balkan Medical Journal. 2013;**30**(1):68-73. DOI: 10.5152/balkanmedj.2012.089

[18] Yildiz S, Gonullu N, Yildiz BP, Hattatoglu DG, Kuskucu M, Midilli K, et al. The role of typical and atypical pathogens in acute exacerbations of chronic obstructive pulmonary disease. The Clinical Respiratory Journal. 2021;**15**(2):209-215. DOI: 10.1111/crj.13286

[19] Aliberti S, Dela Cruz CS, Amati F, Sotgiu G, Restrepo MI. Community-acquired pneumonia. Lancet (London, England). 2021;**398**(10303):906-919. DOI: 10.1016/S0140-6736(21)00630-9

[20] GBD 2016 Lower Respiratory Infections Collaborators. Estimates of the global, regional, and national morbidity, mortality, and aetiologies of lower respiratory infections in 195 countries, 1990-2016: A systematic analysis for the Global Burden of Disease Study 2016. The Lancet. Infectious Diseases. 2018;**18**(11):1191-1210. DOI: 10.1016/S1473-3099(18)30310-4

[21] Heo JY, Song JY. Disease burden and etiologic distribution of community-acquired pneumonia in adults: Evolving epidemiology in the era of pneumococcal conjugate vaccines. Infection and Chemotherapy. 2018;**50**(4):287-300. DOI: 10.3947/ic.2018.50.4.287

[22] Moberg AB, Taléus U, Garvin P, Fransson SG, Falk M. Community-acquired pneumonia in primary care: Clinical assessment and the usability of chest radiography. Scandinavian Journal of Primary Health Care. 2016;**34**(1):21-27. DOI: 10.3109/02813432.2015.1132889

[23] Metlay JP, Waterer GW, Long AC, Anzueto A, Brozek J, Crothers K, et al. Diagnosis and treatment of adults with community-acquired pneumonia. An official clinical practice guideline of the American Thoracic Society and Infectious Diseases Society of America. American Journal of Respiratory and Critical Care Medicine. 2019;**200**(7):e45-e67. DOI: 10.1164/rccm.201908-1581ST

Chapter 6

Challenges of Early Diagnosis and Effective Treatment of Pneumonia in Resource-Limited Settings

Jean-Marie Ntumba Kayembe and Harry-César Ntumba Kayembe

Abstract

Pneumonia is an old known disease but still an health concern, and its burden is differently reported across the world, despite the development of new vaccines and more and more effective antibiotics. Risk factors influencing the outcome of the disease need to be clearly identified, being differently reported between developed versus low-income counties. Demographic data have allowed to illustrate the great vulnerability of patients under five or above sixty-five years old eslsewhere, but les is known about the real impact of socio-economic factors and the impact of environment at the indvidual or community level among people with precarity in low-income countries. There is a great need to determine the role of socio-economic resistance of pathogens to effective antibiotics. To act on modifiable risk factors linked to the human behavior will really help stake holders to address relevant questions in the fight to reduce the burden of morbidity and mortality linked to pneumonia. Diagnosing early and initiating appropriate early treatment is relevant to improve the outcomes of pneumonia elsewhere. Preventive measures need to be directed to socioeconomic backgrounds to act efficiently on the prognosis of respiratory disease.

Keywords: pneumonia, challenges, early diagnosis, treatment, resource-limited settings

1. Introduction

The accurate assessment of incidence of pneumonia worldwide is difficult to reach partially due to the lack of standardized protocols allowing reproducible and regular statistic reporting in many resource-limited settings. According to many previous reports, low tract respiratory infections (LTRI) are described as a leading cause of mortality and morbidity mainly among children under 5 years old and adults above 65 years old, despite the improvement of prevention through vaccination and use of appropriate diagnosis tools and treatment in developed countries [10–13]. Otherwise, mortality due to pneumonia still remains very high in low- and middle-income countries [3, 14, 15]. These observed disparities highlight the need for addressing risk factors of the outcome of CAP to provide adequate preventive and economic healthcare measures. Several hospital–based studies have allowed to identify chronic respiratory diseases and old age as risk factors worsening the prognosis of CAP, along with comorbidities such as cardiovascular or renal diseases, diabetes mellitus, HIV-AIDS, malnitrution and treatment inducing immunosuppression (steroids etc...) [2, 3, 9, 14, 15]. The epidemiological impact of all these conditions need to be clearly established to provide relevant informations in what health measures should be used at individual or community level to reduce the burden of the disease.

The trend in the global incidence of CAP worldwide is always increasing despite vigorous measures developed in many regions of the world [11–13]. Healthcare measures need to relay upon improved knowledge of the impact of socio-demographic elements such as the still great poverty in the sub-Saharan region. Air pollution by impairing the multiple functions of the respiratory system and the climate change through environmental changes could also affect the development of infectious or chronic lung diseases. The real effects of the climate change on the individual and community behavior could alter the environment in a way to weaken some preventive measures. Much has still to be learned on the ecological impact of the climate on the health of human beings and on the behavior of the communities in reaction against the warming temperature. The climate induces environmental changes allowing the emergence of new pathogens worldwide. The real involvement of these ecological modifications needs to be addressed [16–19].

According to the context of occurrence, pneumonia is described as out- or in-hospital. The former is also identified as community-acquired (CAP) and the latter include hospital-acquired or nosocomial pneumonia as well as other forms with different severity levels from really hospital ventilator-acquired or the disease affecting patients in nursing homes or dialysis service [8, 13]. In developing countries, while declining for cardiovascular diseases and cancers, mortality is still static or even rising for CAP [9, 13, 20, 21]. More than 670,000 persons died in 2012 for a respiratory disease in EU representing 13% of all-cause deaths, and pneumonia accounted for 19% among them. Tsoumani et al. reported an incidence of CAP reaching 14 cases/1000 adults in a systematic literature review in Europe with mortality rate of 0.7/1000 cases or 4 million deaths per year [11, 13, 17]. Influenza and CAP are the main providers of death due to infectious origin in this region. In USA, the rate of hospitalization due to pneumonia has fallen from 27% to 23% between 2003 and 2009 with a mortality rate of 22% mainly due to sepsis [22].

Previous systematic analyses for the global burden of disease study estimated yearly deaths in many parts of the world and revealed many epidemiological differences across countries [21, 22]. These studies revealed that an improvement of global life expectancy may be linked to falls in diarrhea, lower tract infections, and neonatal causes in low-income countries and cancer and cardiovascular deaths in developed countries. Many deaths in under five years in children were linked to diarrhea, and malaria, with 2.2 million deaths in 2012, in Nigeria, Democratic Republic of Congo, India, Pakistan, and China [14, 23].

Better understanding of specific risk factors for disease is mandatory for the development of evidence-based recommendations for prevention and treatment.

Data on diagnosis and new emergent risk factors in developing countries are sparse highlighting the need for further researches addressing the main targets for appropriate changes in relevant health policies. There are still many questions requiring urgent responses. This emphasizes the need for targeted researches to identify newer and poorly described relevant factors influencing the prognosis of pneumonia. Despite the development of new antibiotics, outcome of pneumonia is still a health concern, mainly in developing countries. The emerging antibiotic resistance of pathogen appears as a new barrier for relevant health measures in the most affected countries, slowing the infection control worldwide. Innovative approaches through better understanding of clinical features of the disease, the pathophysiology of the related host responses, the environmental changes, the usefulness of modern diagnosis tools to improve early diagnosis, the knowledge of main risk factors and treatment failure need to be developed to improve the control of respiratory mortality. Diagnosis approach of pneumonia relay widely on clinical findings and radiographic evidence of lung consolidations. Laboratory findings depend mainly on the gram stain or culture of sputum or blood culture, with a low sensitivity in determination of the etiologic agent. For this last purpose, new tools of molecular biology are more and more used in developed countries to mitigate this gap; elsewhere, those new tools are out of reach in many poor settings in low- and middle-income countries. Early and sharp diagnosis of infectious diseases is a challenging matter in many parts of the world.

Improving diagnostic approach of pneumonia has to be taken into account the site of infection (out- or in-hospital) and the history of previous acute respiratory infection and antibiotic use with the subsequent risk of emerging resistance, known to interfere with the prognosis. Many pathogens affecting the respiratory tract are airborne-driven, and the hematogenous way may occur, following sepsis; infection could also occur through neighboring contact. The determination of the way of infection onset could guide the empiric choice of the first antibiotic to use during pneumonia, highlighting the relevance of established epidemiologic and environmental data. The environment and the ecology of the pathogens is also very important to consider. To know the evolutionary cycle of the microbe could help in the adoption of preventive measures toward the elimination of intermediate or definitive host concerning emerging and reemerging pathogens as coronaviridae. The One Health strategy includes measures against wildlife and human environment. Climate change and related environment modifications could influence the pathogen ecology and behavior, impairing the host immune responses. The role of social determinants appears more and more important and needs to be clarified in editing prevention methods in the health systems.

It is not often easy to establish the etiological diagnosis of pneumonia; that is a big challenge mainly in middle- and low-income countries. Infectious etiologies include viruses, bacteria, and fungi, requiring costly diagnostic laboratory tools not available at the same level, in all the countries. In Sub-Saharan Africa, many health structures do not have these new opportunities of molecular biology, and clinicians have to develop skills in clinical findings and less sensitivity laboratory tools. This is a very big gap in the decision for empiric antibiotic at the initiation of treatment. Question is about the effectiveness of such therapeutical approach keeping in mind the known variability of etiology with the geographical location. The incidence of pneumonia could also be fueled by the growing market of counterfeit antibiotics widely used in poor-resourced countries subsequent to poor accessibility to effective drugs due to the expensive prices of controlled medicines. It is highly recommended that decision makers provide laws and quality checking laboratories to address the quality of distributed drugs in their countries. Counterfeit trafficking is a great security concern for patients, for the public health system, and the economy in a country. Reviewing the implication of this harmful situation in underdeveloped world is urgently recommended through frequent monitoring measures including health sector, economic, and law administration. Poverty is a leading cause of the failure of health measures in middle-income countries. Pneumonia appear as a disease of poverty, and people are likely to live in overcrowded environment facilitating pneumonia transmission. Poor access to healthcare facilities, lack of modern diagnostic tools for the etiological determination of pathogens, and availability of counterfeit drugs worsen many programs to tackle infectious diseases. The poor compliance to vaccinations due to many wrong beliefs disseminated through social media is a great barrier to the implementation of efficient preventive measures in many underdeveloped countries. No substantial evolution has been made from the 1950s reports, as shown in a recent study from Tanzania highlighting the negative role of epidemiological factors as age and comorbidities and the role of delayed or lack of appropriated diagnosis in the prognosis of CAP [14]. In a systematic analysis for the global burden of disease study 2010, Lozano et al. reported the main role of LTRI ranking fifth in the cause of morbidity and mortality in western regions, while demonstrating the importance of infectious diseases, childhood illnesses, and maternal causes of deaths as major determinants of the burden of the diseases in Sub-Saharan Africa accounting for 70% of all deaths versus 20% in all other countries [22]. The same report identified infectious diseases, childhood illnesses, and maternal causes of death as accounting for 70% of the burden of diseases in sub-Saharan Africa, while representing <20% in all other countries. Low tract respiratory diseases even reduced in developed countries still are classified as big killers globally, causing many early deaths with non-transmissible diseases such as asthma, COPD, and cardiovascular diseases [3, 14, 23].

The variability of pathogen involved in the development of pneumonia and route of entrance in the host's body could influence the outcome of the disease. Some agents are airborne-driven, and others use the hematogenous route. Studies on the ecology of pathogens are needed for relevant therapeutical measures. Viruses are more frequent in cold seasons, while bacteria seem to be more frequent in settings with poor hygiene.

The severity of the disease is also depending on the place of infection onset. Pneumonia is defined as community pneumonia if acquired in the community, out of the hospital. This kind is less severe than hospital-acquired with more probability of resistance to antibiotics. The condition can guide the choice of first-line antibiotics or those with large sensitivity spectrum, as mentioned above. To help make a relevant decision for the treatment of infectious diseases, some conditions need to be met; that is the case of early diagnosis and the identification of the pathogens involved in the development of the disease. The causative agent could be identified through analyses of many specimens, using a lot of technics. Molecular technology as really improved this field, even being not largely available. These molecular approaches are still very expensive and not broadly available in low- and middle-income countries. In the treatment of CAP, the first choice antibiotic should rely on the determination of the etiological pathogen; this goal is not always reachable and the choice usually relies on the knowledge of geographical repartition of the pathogen and the known history of resistance of pathogens to treatment, if available, as well as on the place of occurrence of the disease. This fact highlights the importance of evidence-based studies in this field to improve healthcare decisions at individual or community level. The severity index of the disease from clinical and laboratory indices as well as the comorbidities and availability of effective drugs take an important part in the decision. The knowledge of specific relative risk factors of infectious diseases could really impact on the establishment of relevant prevention or curative health measures and give useful information for treatment decisions.

2. Background

The prognosis of pneumonia is under the influence of many risk factors related to the pathogen and its ecology, to the status of the host, and to environmental issues which need to be clearly understood, to guide relevant health preventive and treatment measures. It is of great relevance to identify these various confounders to help the development of appropriate health policies aiming to reduce the burden of the disease and the still high rate of mortality and morbidity due to this health concern. Early diagnosis and onset of appropriate and effective treatment are among those main determinants of the prognosis. In most low- and middle-income countries, accessibility to modern laboratory tools for etiological diagnosis is limited, and then, early recognition of the disease by health workers in more vulnerable groups remain a big challenge. In these settings, the diagnosis relays upon clinical data and chest X-ray findings where available. Fewer risk factors of poor outcome have been previously described and among them, those linked to the host such as the age under 5 years for children or over 65 years for adults, comorbidities, immunity status, malnutrition, and poverty [1–3]. Less described are the risk factors including the environmental exposure, low social conditions, low salaries, poverty limiting access to health facilities, the role of economic issues such as the growing market of counterfeit drugs; all these emerging factors need to be addressed to provide evidence-based data to improve our knowledge in the implementation of relevant health measures [4–6]. The role of environmental disorders and economic indicators needs to be clarified to guide implementation of health strategies for prevention and effective treatment. Knowledge of geographic repartition of pathogens and epidemiological data of patients are very important in the choice of empiric antibiotic treatment of pneumonia when etiological diagnosis is not available. The seasonal occurrence of viral pneumonia has been reported during winter in many developed countries [7–9], and the role of emerging or reemerging pathogens is a great threat in developing countries with poor access to health facilities. In these countries, the urbanization and industrialization out of the recommended standards facilitate the contact of humans and animals fueling the spread of emerging zoonoses. The relevance of targeted researches in the context of One Health approach appears more and more indicated in infectious diseases control. The environment in which pathogens develop plays a critical role in the occurrence and spread of infectious diseases, such as harmful exposure to outdoor and indoor pollution on respiratory health in vulnerable groups. Global trafficking of counterfeit drugs, mainly antibiotics, is a global threat nowadays, affecting strongly the developing countries, equally more exposed to poverty and lower access to health facilities [4–6]. To what extent precarity linked to bad socio economic conditions could affect the prognosis of infectios diseases meanly in poor ressourced countries need to be carefuly understood for the statement of relevant health measures. Substandard or counterfeit medicines play an important role in the development of pathogen resistance leading to treatment failure and subsequent facilitation of the spread of the disease. The great number of undiagnosed cases or with delayed diagnosis is a great concern where more accurate laboratory tools are not available. This is the case of molecular laboratories using new technologies more expensive in developing countries. The impact of delayed diagnosis on epidemiological and clinical features of the disease has to be clearly determined through evidence-based results to improve health programs for disease control across the world. The link between environmental exposure, social conditions, and population behavior has to be monitored for better specific recommendations. The impact of environmental disorders on respiratory health is far from being clearly understood [9]. It is of relevance to establish the role of the changing environment with industrialization and wild urbanization in low-income countries on the changing behavior of the populations and the health conditions. Despite the development of new antimicrobial drugs, the mortality rate of pneumonia remains high in poor-resourced countries where the delivery of non-controlled medicines is a new challenge to be considered. This phenomenon is empowered by poverty limiting access to appropriate drugs for the management of severe infectious diseases. Inappropriate drug use can lead to resistance to antimicrobial agents and treatment failure with subsequent high rate of mortality. Early diagnosis and onset of the treatment could play a critical role on the control of the disease. Accessibility to appropriate drugs is a challenging matter, being poorer in the underdeveloped countries. To reach the goal of reducing the mortality rate due to pneumonia, it is relevant to address the delayed time to diagnosis, including molecular tools for etiological determination and appropriate management of resistance to anti-microbial agents. The virulence of the pathogen and its immune-evasion capability, a part from acquired resistance to drugs, could negatively influence treatment outcome and need to be considered as indicators of health performances. This chapter addresses above-mentioned risk factors able to worsen the rate of morbidity and mortality due to pneumonia, to provide stakeholders with relevant insights and pivotal recommendations in healthcare decisions. It is a review of the literature through few research motors on the global impact of established and not fully identified prognosis factor for infectious diseases affecting differently the health systems across the world. The chapter aims to sort out the magnitude of deleterious impact of delayed diagnosis and poorness of treatment accessibility on the rate of pneumonia mortality in the developing world, highlighting the importance of holistic approach integrating specific preventive measures, social-based recommendations to tackle poverty, and targeted measures to provide data on the ecology of pathogens to collect evidence-based data for relevant healthcare interventions.

3. Diagnosis of pneumonia

Pneumonia diagnosis rely on clinical features and chest X-ray findings which do not have great sensitivity. Few laboratories could provide etiological informations via Gram stain or culture with limited improvement. The main symptoms such as fever and cough are not disease-specific. The access to chest X-ray examination is also limited to few medical structures in middle- and low-income countries. Etiological diagnosis is not easy, requiring many expensive laboratory tools such as molecular biology, cultures, or more invasive methods, as mentioned above. The empiric antibiotic treatment largely recommended is not the best way to reduce mortality rate.

Despite the development of new antibiotics, the prognosis of CAP remains a great health concern. The improved knowledge of specific risk factor is mandatory to inform health systems. Mortality and morbidity is greatly influenced by demographic factors such as age under five or over 65 years old as previously reported. Air pollution with worsening effects on respiratory system and climate change inducing modifications in the environment are appearing as new conditions needing to be clarified through studies and researches involving multidisciplinary approaches. More vulnerable populations must be determined globally to allow the development of specific and appropriate strategies which could enable the reduction of related morbidity and mortality. It is relevant to learn more about climate changes and induced environmental modifications which worsen the prognosis of airborne-driven diseases and other health concerns such as cancers. In developing countries, populations are exposed to deforestation and not structured urbanization facilitating the neighborhood between humans and animals empowering the emergence of zoonotic diseases due to emerging or re-emerging pathogens such as Ebola virus disease. Many gaps on the knowledge of these less-described risk factors need to be largely addressed to mitigate the impact of diseases in these specific regions. We need to better understand the changing ecology of pathogens and the acquisition of resistance to drugs to improve the efficacy of antimicrobials. There is a great evidence that climate change could impact human being lives showing the relevance of geographic and socioeconomic studies. Poor countries are disproportionately affected compared to developed ones. The relevance of evidence-based data on the deleterious effects of household air quality in many SSA countries has been shown to increase the risk of childhood infectious diseases, highlighting the relevance of researches in this field [16–19]. He et al. reported interactions between environmental factors such as heat, season, and humidity, on the rates of viral infections. It appears more and more clear that the climate should be considered among worsening determinants of the epidemiology of various diseases [17]. Epidemiologic studies in many underdeveloped countries have suggested a possible link between household air pollution and the increasing of the incidence of respiratory diseases [24–26]. Increased risk of pneumonia in children under 5 years has been reported in many parts of this region. This is the case of studies from Ethiopia by Enyew et al., showing an association between the use of biomass and occurrence of acute respiratory infections among children younger than 5 years and a higher prevalence of pneumonia in a same-aged group in East Africa [24] The effect of climate change with warming temperatures and use of wood fires for cooking induce many changes in people behavior and increase the exposition to breathing polluted air. The exposition to poor household air with the cooking habits in many rural areas increasingly impact the health of people by affecting the respiratory health through the development of acute or chronic respiratory disease [25, 26]. The climate change acts through different mechanisms in the increased number of various diseases, acting both on the environment and the host immunity [24–26]. People are thus more exposed to deleterious effects of warming temperatures with an increase in atmospheric ozone, nitrogen oxide, particulate matter (PM), sulfur dioxide, and ultraviolet (UV) radiation. With the increase of temperatures, people are at higher risk of exposition to wild fires, and smoke has deleterious effects on the respiratory functions [25, 26].

According to the infectious agent, its virulence and immunoevasion abilities may influence the outcome of the disease, and host-related factors such as immunity, comorbidities, and aging could also play an important role in the incidence and severity of the illness. Climate change could alter the growth and behavior of pathogens and vectors of zoonotic diseases, thus altering immune reaction of the patient with subsequent worsening of the prognosis impact of the evolution of different diseases [25].

The seasonality of LTRI has been broadly reported, with high incidence during winter in the north regions. In Sub-Saharan regions, respiratory infections are facilitated by many conditions including poverty with limited access to health facilities, air pollution with the use of biomass, and wildfires exposing to inhalation of smoke. Overcrowding creates good conditions for the transmission of airborne pathogens as for pneumonia and TB.

For children under 5 years in low- and middle-income countries, malnutrition with micronutrient deficiency, lack of breastfeeding, the burden of pediatric HIV infection are among the challenging matters worsening the prognosis of infectious diseases [14, 15]. Geography and socio-economic status play a major role in the burden of infectious disease, impacting the lives of people.

The identification of the etiological agents of acute respiratory infection is a great challenge due to the poor sensitivity of microbiological methods and the limited accessibility to culture of respiratory samples. Previous studies place the *Streptococcus pneumoniae* as the more frequent bacteria involved and *Haemophilus influenzae*. Atypical bacteria are more difficult to isolate, the case of *Legionella pneumophila*, Chlamydia, and mycoplasma [10, 13]. Many viruses are also involved in the burden of acute lower respiratory tract infection such as influenza virus, respiratory syncytial virus, rhinovirus, and more others [7, 8].

4. Treatment of pneumonia

The accurate treatment of CAP rely upon the etiological determination, the host status, and also the choice of effective antibiotic in case of bacterial infection. Additional therapeutic measures, such as oxygen therapy are dictated by the existence of comorbidities, the severity of the clinical picture and the involvement of multiple organs. History of pathogen resistance to antibiotic where monitored should guide the first choice antibiotic therapy in suspected bacterial infection. According to the nature of the agent, atypical or typical suspected pneumonia follow some rules for the best treatment to use. B-lactams are widely used alone or associated with macrolides in the former case. CAP could be controlled by oral antibiotics while nosocomial pneumonia could require in-hospital treatment and use of broad spectrum antibiotic. Supportive measures such as oxygen therapy is an option following the severity of the disease. Underlying conditions have to be monitored such as comorbidities. Access to antibiotics is limited in middle- and low-income countries linked to social conditions. People are thus exposed to the market of counterfeit drugs cheaper than accurate ones leading to treatment failure. Guidelines for using severity assessment tools are widely used in developed countries, and they need to be validated in different social and economic conditions in poor-resourced countries.

5. Conclusion

Diagnosing early and initiating appropriate early treatment is relevant to improve the outcomes of pneumonia elsewhere. The inequalities in the development of preventive measures and access to health facilities highlight the need for targeted researches including geographic knowledge of the pathogens, seasonability, and history of previous treatment as well as population characteristics and other specific risk factors in the fight against this leading cause of mortality due to infectious agents. Preventive measures need to be directed to socioeconomic backgrounds to act efficiently on the prognosis of respiratory disease.

Author details

Jean-Marie Ntumba Kayembe[1]* and Harry-César Ntumba Kayembe[2]

1 Service of Respiratory Diseases, Kinshasa University Hospital, DR Congo

2 Department of Basic Sciences, Faculty of Medicine, Kinshasa, DR Congo

*Address all correspondence to: jm.kayembe@unikin.ac.cd

References

[1] Kayembe JMN, Kayembe HCN. Pneumonia: A challenging health concern with the climate change. In: Contempory Topics of Oneumonia. London, UK: Intech; 2017. DOI: 10.5772/intechopen.71609

[2] Wonodi C, Deloria-Knollm M, Feikin DR, et al. Evaluation of risk factors for severe pneumoniain children; the Pneumonia Etiology Research for Child study. Clinical Infectious Diseases. 2012;**54**(Suppl 2):S124-S131

[3] Beletew B, Bimerew M, Mengesha A, et al. Prevalence of pneumonia and its associated factors among under-five children in East Africa: A systematic review and meta-analysis. BMC Pediatrics. 2020;**20**:254

[4] Gautam CS, Utreja A, Singal JL. Spurious and Counterfeit drugs: A growing industry in the developing world. Postgraduate Medical Journal. 2009;**85**(1003):251-256. DOI: 10.1136/pgmj.2008.073213

[5] Tadeg H, Berane Y. Substandard and counterfeit antimicrobials: Recent trends and implications to key public health interventions in developing countries. East African Journal of Public Health. 2012;**9**(2):85-89

[6] Nsimba SE. Counterfeit and substandard drugs in Tanzania: A review. Forensic Science International: Reports. 2022;7(3):100302. DOI: 10.1016/.fsir.2022.100302

[7] Murdoch KM, Mitra B, Lambert S, Erbas B. What is the seasonal distribution of community acquired pneumonia overtime ? A systematic review. Australasian Emergency Nursing Journal. 2014;**17**:30-42

[8] Chalmers JD, Plet MW, Alibert S. Community-Acquired Pneumonia, European Respiratory Monographs. Sheffield: European Respiratory Society; 2014. ISBN: 978-1-849-84049-1

[9] Gibson GJ, Loddenkemper R, Lundba B, Sibille Y. Respiratory health and disease in Europe: The new European Lung White Book. European Respiratory Journal. 2013;**42**:559-563. DOI: 10.1183/09031936.00105513

[10] Gilani Z, Kwong YD, Levine OS, et al. A literature review and survey of survey of childhood pneumonia etiologystudies: 2000-2010. Clinical Infectious Diseases. 2012;**54**(Suppl 2):S102-S108

[11] Torres A, Peetermans E, Viegi G, Biasi F, et al. Risk factors for community-acquired pneumoniain adults in Europe: A literature rewiew. Thorax. 2013;**68**:1057-1065. DOI: 1136/thoraxjnl-2013

[12] Welte T, Torres A, Nathwani D. Clinical and economic burden of community-acquired pneumonia among adults in Europe. Thorax. 2012;**67**(1):71-79. DOI: 10.111136/thx.2009.129502

[13] Tsoumani E, Carter JA, Salomonsson S, Stephens JM, Bencina G, et al. Clinical, economic, and humanistic burden of community acquired pneumonia in Europe: A systematic literature review. Expert Review of Vaccines. 2023;**22**(1):876-884

[14] Caggiano S, Ullmann N, De Vitis E, Trivelli M, Mariani C, Podagrosi M, et al. Factors that negatively affect the prognosis of pediatric community-acquired pneumonia in district hospital in Tanzania. International Journal

of Molecular Sciences. 2017;**18**:3. DOI: 10.3390/ijms18030623

[15] Gray DM, Hj Z. Community-acquired pneumonia in HIV-infected children: A global perspective. Current Opinion in Pulmonary Medicine. 2010;**16**:208-216

[16] Joshi M, Joshi A, barter T. Climate change and respiratory diseases: A 2020 perspective. Current Opinion in Pulmonary Medicine. 2020;**26**:119-127

[17] He Y, Liu WJ, Jia N, et al. Viral respiratory infections in a rapidly changing climate: The need to prepare for the next pandemic. eBioMedicine. 2023;**93**:104593

[18] Dobson A. Climate variability, global change, immunity, and the dynamics of infectious diseases. Ecology. 2009;**90**:920-927

[19] Romanello M, Di Napoli C, Drummond P. The 2023 report of the Lancet Countdown on health and climate change: The imperative for a health-centred response in a world facing irreversible harms. Lancet. 2022;**400**:1619-1654

[20] Lindenauer PK, Lagu T, Shieh MS, et al. Association of diagnostic coding with trends in hospitalizations and mortality of patients with pneumonia 2003-2009. JAMA. 2012;**307**:1405-1413

[21] GBD Collaborators. Global, regional and national levels of age-specific mortality and 240 causes of death, 1990-2013: A systematic analysis for the Global burden of Disease Study 2013. Lancet. 2015;**385**:1990-2013

[22] Lozano R, Naghavi M, Foreman K, et al. Global and regional mortality from 235 causes of death for 20 age groups in 1990 and 2010: A systematic analysis for the global burden of disease study 2010. Lancet. 2012;**380**(9859):2095-2128

[23] Theodoratou E, Al-Jilaih S, Woodward T, et al. The effect of case management on childhood pneumonia mortality in developing countries. International Journal of Epidemiology. 2010;**39**(Suppl. 1):i155-i171

[24] Enyew HD, Mereta ST, Hailu AB. Biomass fuel use and acute respiratory infection among children younger than 5 years in Ethiopia: A systematic review and meta-analysis. Public Health. 2021;**193**:29-40

[25] Mirsaeidi M, Motahari H, Khamesi MT, Sharif A, Campos M, Schraufnagel DE. Climate change and respiratory infections. Annals of the American Thoracic Society. 2016;**13**(8):1223-1230. DOI: 10.1513/AnnalsATS.201511-729PS

[26] Woolley KE, Bagambe T, Singh A, et al. Investigating the association between wood and charcoal domestic cooking, respiratory symptoms and acute respiratory infections among children aged under 5 years in Uganda: A cross-sectional analysis of the 2016 demographic and health survey. International Journal of Environmental Research and Public Health. 2020;**17**:3974

Section 5

Foundations of Virology and Global Health Perspectives Including Regional Insights

Chapter 7

Emerging and Re-Emerging Viral Infections: Trends in Africa

Prince Amoah Barnie, Evans Tumawu, Festus Agbatey, Godwin Amponsah Asiamah, William Gyamesi, Karen Pomeyie and Helena Quayson

Abstract

The emergence and reemergence of viral infections pose significant public health challenges in Africa. This narrative review examines the trends, epidemiology, and contributing factors behind viral outbreaks on the continent. The review highlights major viral diseases such as Ebola, Lassa fever, monkeypox, Rift Valley fever, and COVID-19, emphasizing their impact on morbidity and mortality. Key drivers of viral emergence include ecological disruption, human behavioral factors, globalization, and viral genetic evolution. The chapter also explores regional distribution patterns, with Ebola and Lassa fever predominantly affecting West Africa, while monkeypox and Marburg virus disease remain concerns in Central Africa. Additionally, vector-borne infections such as dengue, chikungunya, and yellow fever persist in East and West Africa. Public health strategies to mitigate viral threats involve integrated surveillance systems, the One Health approach, vaccine deployment, and vector control measures. However, challenges such as weak healthcare infrastructure, limited genomic surveillance, and vaccine inequity hinder effective disease control. This underscores the need for strengthened pandemic preparedness, improved disease monitoring, and multidisciplinary collaborations to curb future outbreaks. Addressing these challenges through sustained investment in public health infrastructure and international cooperation is essential to safeguarding African populations against emerging and reemerging viral infections.

Keywords: emerging viruses, remerging viruses, viral infections, Africa, trends

1. Introduction

Africa, a vast continent made up of 54 nations, including several island states, has reported numerous vector-borne and zoonotic viral diseases across different regions [1].

The outbreak of coronavirus (SARS-CoV-2) in China in December 2019 led to the emergence of COVID-19 in humans. Additionally, the spread of Ebola virus disease (EVD), Marburg virus disease, monkeypox virus disease, and dengue fever in Africa has underscored the critical importance of zoonotic viral diseases in Africa. The emergence and reemergence of viral infections have become a public health concern in recent times. At a basic level, an emerging viral infection can be defined as a newly identified infection that is increasing within a population or has experienced a rise in occurrence or spread to new geographic regions, hosts, or vectors [2], while the reemerging viral infection is defined as an infection that resurfaces after having been largely controlled [3]. However, population growth, poverty, malnutrition, increased domestic and international travel, economic pressures that drive migration, social behaviors, the spread of immunosuppressive diseases, unplanned urbanization, deforestation, and changes in agricultural practices like mixed farming are some of the factors that contribute to the emergence and reemergence of these infections [4]. Regrettably, many of these factors are disproportionately prevalent in numerous African countries.

The emergence and re-emergence of viral infections have been associated with high mortality rates in Africa [5]. The Ebola virus outbreak in West Africa is reported to have resulted in over 11,000 deaths between 2013 and 2016 [6]. More recently, the SARS-CoV-2 infection has led to 257,984 deaths in Africa [2]. In addition, meningitis, measles, yellow fever, monkeypox, Zika, Rift Valley fever, dengue fever, and Marburg virus disease are among the newly discovered infectious diseases that have been linked to high mortality rates in Africa [7].

Approximately 60% of infectious diseases and 75% of newly discovered human infections are zoonotic, with two-thirds originating from wildlife [8]. Zoonotic diseases are infections that are passed from vertebrates to humans [9]. Zoonotic diseases have disproportionately impacted vulnerable populations in Africa and have often been 'neglected' due to the political tension and the funding allocated for the prevention, control, and research [10, 11]. Access to technologies is still limited in Africa, despite advancements in disease monitoring, such as the use of genetic epidemiology methods during recent Ebola outbreaks in Guinea and the Democratic Republic of the Congo [12, 13]. However, unplanned urbanization has led to habitat destruction, drawing humans closer into contact with animals and arthropod vectors of viral infections. As a result, these interactions have significantly contributed to the rise in human vulnerability to infections by new pathogens, particularly in the immunocompromised and impoverished population [3].

Public health strategies aimed at controlling emerging viral infections emphasize integrated one-health approaches, which incorporate human, animal, and environmental health perspectives [14, 15]. Several studies highlight the importance of multisectoral collaborations in establishing effective surveillance systems, though institutional and logistical barriers persist in Africa [16–18]. In addition, vaccine deployment and strategies for vector control are fundamental to curbing the spread of infections, yet challenges such as vaccine inequities and insecticide resistance undermine their effectiveness [19]. The COVID-19 pandemic has emphasized the necessity to enhance genomic surveillance, early warning systems, and pandemic preparedness policies tailored to African public health infrastructures [12, 20]. This chapter explores the trends of emerging and reemerging viral infections in Africa by examining recent literature to assess the predominant trends, influencing factors, and strategies for addressing emerging and reemerging viral infections in Africa.

2. Methodology

This narrative review was conducted to synthesize the trends of emerging and re-emerging viral infections in Africa. A thorough literature search was performed using PubMed, ScienceDirect, CDC, and WHO repositories, focusing on articles published from 2000 to 2024. The following keywords and Boolean combinations were used to identify relevant studies: "emerging viral infections", "trends", "viral evolution," "re-emerging viral diseases," "emerging viral infections" vs. "re-emerging viral diseases," ("drivers OR determinants") AND "viral evolution," and ("emerging viral infections" OR "re-emerging viral diseases") AND Africa.

2.1 Notable emerging/reemerging viral infections in Africa

Many viruses, some of which are in **Table 1**, have appeared or resurfaced in human populations during the last 50 years. The table highlights notable viruses that have emerged in Africa recently.

Viral infection	Viral name	Reservoir/ vector	Year of first detection	Significant outbreaks
Chikungunya fever	Chikungunya virus	Mosquito	1824, India [21]	India and Sri Lanka in 1962. Over 200 deaths [22]
Covid-19	*SARS-CoV-2*	Bats	December 2019 [23]	2019–2022 Over 9 million cases as of June 2020 [24]
Dengue Fever	Dengue virus	Mosquito	Over 200 years ago [25].	2017–2018 400 confirmed cases
Ebola virus disease (EVD)	Ebola virus	Bats	1976, Sudan and Dr. Congo [26]	2014 outbreak in Guinea, Sierra Leone, and Liberia [27]
Monkeypox	Monkeypox virus	Rodent	1958, Denmark [28]	2022 outbreak [29]
Marburg virus disease (MVD)	Marburg virus	Fruit bat	1967 [30]	1998–2000 outbreak, Angola [31]
Lassa Fever	Lassa virus	Rodent	1969, Nigeria [32]	2017–2018 Outbreak 400 confirmed cases [33].
Zika virus	Zika virus	Mosquito	1947, Uganda and Tanzania [34]	

Table 1.
Examples of recent viral infection outbreaks, zoonosis, and other notable infectious disease events in Africa.

3. Epidemiological trends and geographic distribution of viral infections in Africa

The distribution of viral infections across different regions of Africa is influenced by various ecological, socio-economic, and healthcare-related factors [14]. The WHO African Region, home to about 1.1 billion people, representing 14% of the global population, consists of 47 diverse member states. Despite notable advancements in viral disease infection management, the region continues to face significant health and socioeconomic challenges due to an unequal disease burden relative to its population size. Over the past two decades, life expectancy and healthy life expectancy have generally improved across the region. However, available data indicate that the COVID-19 pandemic, Ebola virus, and other viral infections have hindered progress toward achieving the Sustainable Development Goals (SDGs) [35]. Some viral infections are endemic to specific regions, while others have exhibited widespread transmission across Africa. The emergence and re-emergence of these infections, particularly in tropical, subtropical, and developing African countries, highlight the ongoing public health challenges they pose [36]. The distribution of viral infection across Africa is discussed in detail in the following sections.

3.1 West Africa: Ebola, Lassa fever, yellow fever

West Africa is a hotspot for viral hemorrhagic fevers, such as yellow fever, Lassa fever, and Ebola. The Ebola virus, first discovered in 1976, resurged in the 2014–2016 outbreak, which primarily affected Guinea, Sierra Leone, Nigeria, Senegal, and Mali [37]. The first outbreak of this viral infection in West Africa was observed in Guinea in December 2013. The Ebola virus has emerged sporadically across Africa, causing outbreaks ranging from small to large scale. The World Health Organization (WHO) recorded 3444 cases during the ongoing Ebola outbreak in the Democratic Republic of the Congo in 2020, which included 3310 confirmed cases and 134 suspected cases, resulting in 2264 recorded deaths from the confirmed cases and a very high mortality rate of 65.74% [38]. Studies on various animal species during an Ebola virus disease (EVD) outbreak have identified certain species of fruit bats as likely reservoirs of the virus [39]. The mode of transmission is through direct contact with blood, body fluids, and secretions [39]. The Zaire, Sudan, Ivory Coast, and Bundibugyo Ebola Viruses are the four African strains of the Ebola virus that have been previously discovered in Africa [40].

Lassa fever, endemic to Nigeria and surrounding countries, is transmitted through rodent exposure [41]. This zoonotic acute viral hemorrhagic fever (VHF) is caused by a single-stranded RNA virus that is a member of the Arenaviridae family [42]. It is estimated to cause about two million infections, with 300,000 to 500,000 clinical cases and 10,000 deaths annually among people in the West African sub-region [43]. In Nigeria, Outbreaks of Lassa fever often peak in severity from the last quarter of the year to the first quarter of the following year, after which cases decline for the rest of the year. This pattern is largely attributed to a rise in rodent populations, driven by favorable breeding conditions toward the end of the rainy season and the start of the dry season, when food is more abundant on farms [44, 45].

Yellow fever, a mosquito-borne flavivirus, remains a concern despite vaccination efforts, with periodic outbreaks in countries like Nigeria and Ghana [46]. The World Health Organization (WHO) receives reports of at least one yellow fever (YF) outbreak each year in Africa; over the past 15 years, its incidence has been gradually rising [47]. The yellow fever virus is spread by female Aedes mosquitoes between vertebrate hosts. According to Findlay et al. [48], yellow fever has been circulating in the regions of Africa. The World Health Organization (WHO) currently defines the yellow fever (YF) endemic region in Africa as spanning approximately 15° north and 15° south of the equator, as shown in **Figure 1**. This area covers 34 African countries, stretching from the southern boundary of Angola in the south to the Sahara Desert in the north. It is home to nearly 500 million people, all of whom are susceptible to contracting yellow fever (YF). There are three primary climate zones in the African region where yellow fever is endemic: The Moist Savanna, which is outside the rainforest and is distinguished by progressively declining rainfall, is part of the Equatorial Rainforest, which stretches from Guinea in West Africa to western Uganda in East Africa and as far south as northern Angola. Often referred to as the "zone of emergence," it is a significant agricultural hub and the source of numerous YF outbreaks. Dry Savanna, which is located further out from the wet savanna, has even less rainfall and is the periphery of the YF-endemic zone.

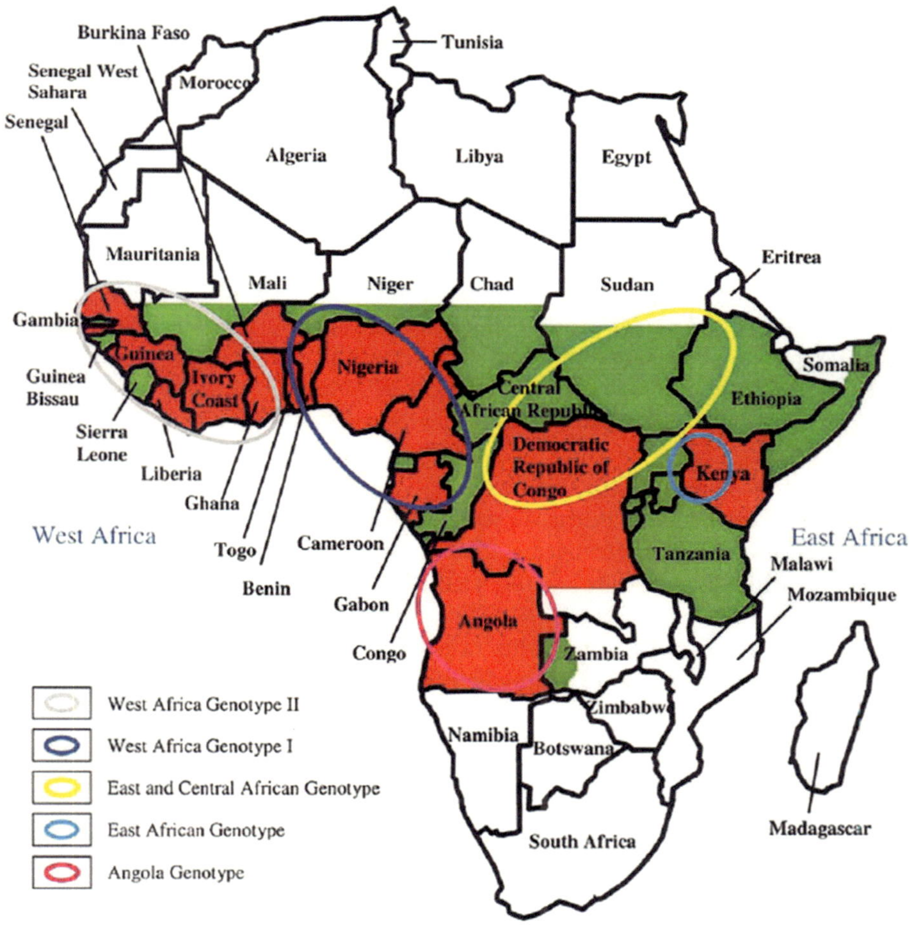

Figure 1.
A map of Africa that shows the designated distribution of YF genotypes (shown as coloured ellipses) and the endemic area of YF (shown in red and green). According to WHO data, the countries shown in red are those that reported YF epidemics between 1984 and 2001 [49].

3.2 Central Africa: Monkeypox and Ebola

Central Africa continues to experience outbreaks of monkeypox and Ebola. The epicenter of the Monkeypox virus disease is the Democratic Republic of the Congo (DRC), with frequent outbreaks due to human-wildlife interactions and weak health-care infrastructure [50]. Monkeypox, a zoonotic viral disease related to smallpox, has seen increased incidence in the DRC and Cameroon, often linked to animal reservoirs and declining smallpox immunity [51]. The first reported case of Monkeypox in Africa was in the Democratic Republic of Congo (DRC) in 1970 [52]. On August 14, 2024, the increase in monkey pox cases in the Democratic Republic of the Congo and its increasing spread to Burundi, Kenya, Rwanda, Uganda, Ghana, and Côte d'Ivoire were emphasized by the WHO Director-General [53]. The monkeypox virus has been spreading rapidly among adults through close physical contact, including sexual transmission within networks such as sex workers and clients. As the virus continues to spread, the affected populations are shifting, with transmission now occurring within households and other community settings [53]. However, between 2022 and 2024, a total of 45,652 monkeypox cases with laboratory and clinical confirmation occurred in 12 African nations, resulting in 1492 fatalities and a 3.3% case fatality rate based on laboratory-confirmed cases [54]. Central and Western Africa recorded the majority of the cases reported. In Côte d'Ivoire, consuming monkeys as a delicacy is a common practice in regions prone to Monkeypox outbreaks. This, along with activities such as hunting and butchering, may serve as a significant source of disease transmission [55].

3.3 East Africa: Rift valley fever, dengue, and chikungunya

East Africa is prone to arboviral dengue, chikungunya, and Rift Valley fever. Rift Valley fever (RVF), primarily affecting Kenya and Tanzania, is spread by mosquitoes, and it endangers both human and livestock populations, particularly during heavy rainfall [56]. Dengue and chikungunya, spread by Aedes mosquitoes, have been reported in Somalia, Sudan, and Kenya, exacerbated by urbanization and climate change [57]. Dengue fever impacts around 400 million people globally each year, leading to approximately 22,000 fatalities [58]. The death rate of dengue fever in Africa varies by country and outbreak severity. Current World Health Organization (WHO) data shows that, in Mauritius, there have been 2534 reported cases in 2024, with three deaths, Côte d'Ivoire has reported 325 confirmed cases with three deaths, resulting in a death rate of about 0.6%, Ethiopia, 17 deaths have been reported out of 23,277 cases, leading in a case fatality rate (CFR) of 0.07%, Mali and Cabo Verde have reported no deaths despite having 229 confirmed cases and 543 confirmed cases, respectively [59].

The Chikungunya virus (CHIKV) re-emerged along the eastern coast of Africa between 2004 and 2005, affecting regions like Lamu and Madagascar [36]. The virus can infect a significant portion of the population in a few short weeks [60]. It is thought that CHIKV causes more symptomatic infections than other arboviral illnesses.

3.4 Southern Africa: HIV/AIDS

Southern Africa has the highest burden of HIV/AIDS globally, particularly in South Africa, Eswatini, and Botswana, where incident rates exceed 20% in some populations [61]. However, in a recent report, approximately 25.6 million people in Africa were infected with HIV, highlighting the ongoing need for efforts to curb the disease's spread. Eastern and Southern Africa accounted for around 20.8 million of these cases, while West and Central Africa contributed nearly 4.8 million new infections. As a result, over half of the global HIV infections that year originated in sub-Saharan Africa [62]. Transferring body fluids from an infected individual, such as blood, breast milk, semen, and vaginal secretions, can spread HIV. However, commonplace activities like kissing, hugging, handshakes, and sharing food, water, or personal belongings cannot spread it [63].

3.5 North Africa: Hepatitis

North Africa experiences high hepatitis prevalence, particularly hepatitis C (HCV), which is endemic in Egypt due to past unsafe medical practices [64]. Egypt thus has the world's highest prevalence of HCV [65]. In Africa, more than 91 million people are affected by hepatitis B or C, representing 26% of the worldwide burden of these infections and leading to approximately 125,000 deaths each year [66]. Several factors contribute to the risk of HCV infection in Africa, these include traditional practices such as geographical location, unsafe blood transfusions, inappropriate injectable drug usage, scarification, a family history of viral hepatitis, and high-risk sexual behaviors involving blood exposure [67]. Aside from HCV being highly prevalent in Egypt, other countries such as the Democratic Republic of the Congo, Nigeria, Cameroon, Gabon, and Libya have also notably recorded high prevalence rates [68]. The variation in prevalence figures reported by different studies within the same region highlights the challenges associated with epidemiological surveillance.

4. Factors driving viral emergence and reemergence in Africa

Viral Infectious diseases emerge and re-emerge over time. Before causing an outbreak, pathogens undergo various adaptation stages to adjust to a new host [69]. The emergence and reemergence of infectious diseases are heavily influenced by the complex interactions between pathogens, hosts, and environmental conditions. Ecological, environmental, and demographic factors significantly shape these adaptations, often increasing exposure to previously unfamiliar pathogens or their natural hosts and aiding their transmission [70]. In Africa, three major factors drive viral emergence and reemergence: Ecological Disruption, Human Factors, and Viral Factors.

4.1 Human factors

The emergence and reemergence of viral illnesses are significantly influenced by a wide range of factors related to human behavior and societal structures. The rapid migration from rural to urban areas has led to the growth of high-density peri-urban slums, creating ideal conditions for vector breeding. Unplanned urbanization is often characterized by inadequate housing and a lack of essential services, such as clean water and proper waste management, further supporting the expansion of vector populations. As urbanization increases, the concentration of people in cities and towns results in overcrowded environments, making the spread of infectious diseases more likely, particularly in places with inadequate access to clean water and poor sanitation [71]. According to Pearce et al. [72], urbanization can create diverse interactions between wildlife, livestock, and humans, serving as a critical point for both the emergence of new pathogens and the transmission of diseases across species.

In Africa, certain human lifestyle choices, like sexual activities, body modifications like tattoos and piercings, and intravenous drug use, contribute to the spread of viruses such as hepatitis and HIV [73]. According to Guure et al. [74], the use of intravenous drugs like heroin, crack, cocaine, and tramadol exposed people to infections caused by hepatitis B, C, and HIV. Religious and spiritual practices can also influence disease transmission. According to Manguvo and Mafuvadze [75], the handling and touching of deceased people have been implicated in the transmission of Ebola viruses, while outbreaks of polio and measles frequently take place in religious groups that oppose immunizations. Similarly, the spread of monkeypox among people in central and western Africa is due to deforestation [76]. As human settlements expand into rainforest edges and encroach on forested areas, individuals come into contact with infected rodents native to these environments. Monkeypox is primarily spread to humans through contact with an animal's blood or by rodent bites from infected rodents [76].

Finally, the consumption of partially prepared foods creates opportunities for the transmission of foodborne viruses such as hepatitis A. A recent study found that the virus can remain infectious for several days on fruits and vegetables, which are commonly eaten raw or undercooked. These imported products have already been linked to disease outbreaks [77].

4.2 Ecological disruption

Disease emergence can also be significantly influenced by a region's natural features. By changing natural ecosystems, environmental disturbances like pollution and deforestation might increase viral exposure [78]. According to Alexander et al. [79], the outbreak of the Ebola virus in West Africa has been linked to deforestation, which led to the destruction of vital habitats for fruit bats. In another study, deforestation has been associated with the re-emergence of the Nipah virus in Malaysia and Singapore [80, 81].

Agricultural development, a common way humans modify and interact with the environment, often contributes to the emergence of diseases. Hantaan virus, responsible for the Korean hemorrhagic fever, is reported to naturally infect the rice-field-dwelling field mouse Apodemus agrarius. Humans typically contract the disease during the rice harvest through exposure to infected rodents [82]. Similarly, increased contact with pig farms has been linked to the resurgence of the Rift Valley fever virus, which led to outbreaks in Kenya in 2006 and Sudan in 2007, as well as in Saudi Arabia in 2000 [83, 84]. Again, data show that over 50% of newly discovered zoonotic illnesses in humans and over 25% of newly discovered infectious diseases are caused by agricultural causes [85].

4.3 Viral factors

Viruses, like all other living things, are constantly evolving. Numerous viruses exhibit a high mutation rate, allowing them to evolve quickly and produce new variants. A well-known example is antigenic drift in influenza. Similarly, the SARS coronavirus likely underwent genetic modifications, including a 29-base deletion, as it spread from its original host to humans. Although the impact of these genetic changes remains uncertain, they may have contributed to the increased transmissibility of the virus among humans.

RNA viruses make up the majority of the viral agents in newly emerging and re-emerging infectious diseases [86]. RNA viruses have a high mutation rate due to the low accuracy of RNA-dependent RNA polymerase, which lacks proofreading capabilities, and the error-prone reverse transcriptase (RT) used by retroviruses, both of which do not possess the 3′ → 5′ exonuclease activity necessary for error correction, contributing to viral diversity [87]. This leads to high mutation rates and genetic recombination, enabling RNA viruses to adapt to environmental changes and host immune responses. The genetic variants of the viral genome that cause the virus to evolve quickly and adapt to its environment are point mutation, recombination, and reassortment [88]. Among these, the most used adaptation technique for virus evolution is point mutation [87]. Key antigenic regions in influenza A virus are altered by the slow accumulation of point mutations in the hemagglutinin (HA) surface glycoprotein. These modifications enable the virus to evade recognition by antibodies produced from previous infections, a process known as "antigenic drift," which contributes to ongoing seasonal outbreaks [89].

However, viruses create new "hybrid" or "mixed" genomes through recombination, which is the exchange of genetic material between two copies [90]. A report shows that (1) large genome size, (2) discontinuous transcription, and (3) the presence of both full-length and sub-genomic RNAs, which provide more templates for strand switching, are the factors that contributed to the high recombination rates in these viruses [30].

Finally, gene reassortment is the third viral adaptation of the virus. This occurs in segmented viruses, which possess multiple genome segments. The exchange of genome segments between two or more viruses that co-infect the same cell can produce offspring viruses that have genetic material from several parent viruses. According to Domingo [87], this mechanism is implicated in the influenza A virus genome consisting of eight segments of ssRNA.

5. Future perspective

Although viral infection emergence or reemergence is challenging, it is possible to strengthen infrastructure and implement broad measures to enhance public health systems and improve population preparedness for future infectious disease outbreaks. A significant obstacle in controlling viral infection arises from their transmission being largely influenced by wildlife reservoirs. As a result, prevention efforts that focus solely on either human or animal health are often ineffective [91]. The following strategies have been identified as appropriate and effective for managing zoonotic viral diseases.

5.1 Surveillance

Epidemiological surveillance is one of the core measures that should be taken to manage viral infection in Africa. Detecting a new viral disease requires surveillance systems that track routine cases and identify irregularities when unusual patterns emerge [92]. To accomplish this, regular testing of both humans and animals is essential to detect disease agents before epidemics arise. Given the modern rise of viral infection across Africa, it is possible that infected individuals and vectors were transported from one African country to another. For instance, the introduction of Rift Valley fever into Egypt in 1977 and the Arabian Peninsula in 2000 occurred following outbreaks in Sudan in 1976 and the Horn of Africa in 1998 [93, 94].

Implementing effective disease surveillance in Africa remains difficult, particularly in remote rural areas with limited transportation networks. Research in Zambia, for instance, highlighted inadequate transport infrastructure as a major barrier to successfully executing a comprehensive disease monitoring and response system [95]. Similar to this, a review study finds that transport is one of the major obstacles to surveillance in Africa, along with non-sustainable financial resources, poor coordination, insufficient training and turnover of peripheral staff, inconsistent feedback, insufficient supervision from the next level, and weak laboratory capacities [96]. A recent study further illustrated this issue by showing that enhancements in transportation infrastructure in Uganda in 2016 led to more effective case reporting, thereby strengthening disease surveillance efforts [97]. Epidemiological surveillance during an outbreak can generate valuable data that helps assess and enhance public health and medical response efforts in times of viral infection.

5.2 Implementation of one health

The One Health approach is increasingly recognized as the best method for dealing with new risks of infectious diseases [98]. The foundation of the One Health idea is the knowledge that environmental, animal, and human health are interrelated. It acknowledges that animal species serve as a common reservoir for pathogen transmission and that numerous emerging infectious diseases (EIDs) are influenced by diverse and evolving animal- human interactions [99]. The emergence and re-emergence of viral infections in Africa are defined by their complexity and the uncertainty surrounding their causes, impacts, and potential solutions [100]. In Africa, the emergence and cross-species transmission of many pathogens, such as Ebola virus disease (EVD), Marburg virus disease, monkeypox virus, and dengue fever, are largely driven by human activities, including deforestation, agricultural expansion, increased global trade and travel, and the intensification of animal farming [101–103]. The rapid advancements in our knowledge of the biology and epidemiology of these viruses highlight the significant improvements in responding to emerging infectious disease threats over recent decades. However, emerging and reemerging viral infections continue to represent a serious threat to public health and community well-being throughout the continent, despite improvements in diagnostics, therapies, and vaccine development brought about by advances in immunobiology and genetics.

Emerging infectious disease (EID) threats persist despite scientific advances, as they are not solely caused by pathogens crossing species barriers. Instead, they stem from intricate and interdependent factors, including socioeconomic and sociopolitical influences, which extend beyond the direct impact of the disease itself. The successful practical implementation of the One Health approach in Africa can help mitigate EID. The One Health implementation involves key strategies, such as the integrated surveillance systems, cross-sectoral collaboration, community engagement, and education and policy and legislation.

5.2.1 Integrated surveillance systems

Coordinated monitoring of wildlife, livestock, and human populations is essential for the early detection of emerging pathogens [104]. According to WHO, the consequences extend beyond nature when animals fall ill or die in the wild; 75% of emerging human infections originate from animals. Disease outbreaks like avian influenza, SARS, and COVID-19 have demonstrated how viruses can transfer from animals to humans, leading to worldwide crises [105]. Surveillance programs such as the Global Early Warning System (GLEWS) facilitate timely identification and response to zoonotic threats.

5.2.2 Cross-sectoral collaboration

Partnerships between medical professionals, veterinarians, ecologists, and policymakers enhance disease outbreak preparedness and response [106]. The One Health approach promotes collaborative research by uniting experts from various fields to address complex health challenges. For example, interdisciplinary teams examining zoonotic diseases can explore ecological influences, animal hosts, and human interactions that drive disease transmission. This comprehensive strategy enhances the understanding of disease patterns and supports the development of effective prevention and control measures [107]. Such cooperation is actively encouraged by agencies such as the World Health Organization (WHO), the Food and Agriculture Organization (FAO), and the World Organization for Animal Health (OIE).

5.2.3 Community engagement and education

Public awareness campaigns are crucial in encouraging preventive measures such as proper sanitation, vaccination, and responsible animal husbandry practices [108]. Engaging local communities in disease prevention efforts strengthens public health responses. A study revealed that a straightforward awareness campaign successfully enhanced knowledge of rabies symptoms and vaccination schedules. Notably, individuals exposed to the campaign were 1.4 times more likely to report vaccinating their pets, a critical measure in preventing human rabies [109].

5.2.4 Policy and legislation

One Health advocates for policies that acknowledge the connection between environmental, animal, and human health. These policies should encourage cross-sector collaboration and coordination to tackle health challenges more efficiently [110]. For instance, adopting integrated water management strategies can help minimize the risk of waterborne diseases, improving health outcomes for both humans and animals. [111]. Again, policies that enforce biosecurity measures and restrict illegal wildlife trade, serve as a significant pathway for zoonotic spillovers [112]. Policies guided by the One Health approach promote sustainable agriculture and the prudent use of antimicrobials, safeguarding the long-term health of ecosystems and communities [113].

6. Conclusion

The emergence and reemergence of viral infections in Africa pose significant public health challenges, influenced by factors such as ecological disruptions, human activities, and viral evolution. The continent has experienced recurrent outbreaks of zoonotic diseases, including Ebola, Lassa fever, monkeypox, and Rift Valley fever, often exacerbated by environmental changes and inadequate healthcare infrastructure. Additionally, vector-borne diseases like dengue, chikungunya, and yellow fever continue to burden populations, while chronic infections such as HIV/AIDS and hepatitis remain persistent threats. Addressing these challenges requires a comprehensive and multidisciplinary approach, integrating epidemiological surveillance, vaccine deployment, vector control strategies, and the One Health framework, which emphasizes collaboration between human, animal, and environmental health sectors. Strengthening healthcare systems, improving disease monitoring, and fostering community awareness are essential steps toward mitigating future outbreaks. Although scientific advancements in genomics, diagnostics, and vaccine development have improved disease preparedness and response, gaps remain in research funding, healthcare accessibility, and policy implementation. Tackling emerging and reemerging viral infections in Africa demands sustained investment in public health infrastructure, international cooperation, and proactive policies to prevent future epidemics. By prioritizing early detection, rapid response strategies, and innovative research, Africa can better manage viral threats and safeguard its populations from devastating outbreaks.

Emerging and Re-Emerging Viral Infections: Trends in Africa
DOI: http://dx.doi.org/10.5772/intechopen.1014144

Author details

Prince Amoah Barnie[1,2,3*], Evans Tumawu[4], Festus Agbatey[1], Godwin Amponsah Asiamah[1], William Gyamesi[1], Karen Pomeyie[5,6] and Helena Quayson[5]

1 Department of Forensic Sciences, School of Biological Sciences, University of Cape Coast, Ghana

2 International Genome Centre, Jiangsu University, Zhenjiang, Jiangsu Province, P.R. China

3 Department of Immunology, Jiangsu University, Zhenjiang, Jiangsu Province, P.R. China

4 Department of Biomedical Sciences, School of Allied Health Sciences, University of Cape Coast, Ghana

5 Department of Microbiology and Immunology, School of Medical Sciences, University of Cape Coast, Ghana

6 Department of Virology, Noguchi Memorial Institute for Medical Research, College of Health Sciences, University of Ghana, Ghana

*Address all correspondence to: pamoah-barnie@ucc.edu.gh

References

[1] Ndembi N, Yumo H, Takehisa J, Takemura T, Kobayashi E, Ngansop C, et al. HIV type 1 infection in pygmy hunter gatherers is from contact with bantu rather than from nonhuman primates. AIDS Research and Human Retroviruses. 2003;**19**(5):435-439. DOI: 10.1089/088922203765551773

[2] WHO. Report of the WHO/FAO/OIE joint consultation on emerging zoonotic diseases/in collaboration with the Health Council of the Netherlands; 2023

[3] Mourya DT, Yadav PD, Ullas PT, Bhardwaj SD, Sahay RR, Chadha MS, et al. Emerging/re-emerging viral diseases & new viruses on the Indian horizon. Indian Journal of Medical Research. 2019;**149**(4):447-467. DOI: 10.4103/ijmr.IJMR_1239_18

[4] Mani RS, Ravi V, Desai A, Madhusudana S. Emerging viral infections in India. Proceedings of the National Academy of Sciences, India Section B: Biological Sciences. 2012;**82**:5-21. DOI: 10.1007/s40011-011-0001-1

[5] Fenollar F, Mediannikov O. Emerging infectious diseases in Africa in the 21st century. New Microbes and New Infections. 2018;**26**:S10-S18. DOI: 10.1016/j.nmni.2018.09.004

[6] Jacob ST, Crozier I, Fischer WA, Hewlett A, Kraft CS, Vega M-A d L, et al. Ebola virus disease. Nature Reviews Disease Primers. 2020;**6**(1):13. DOI: 10.1038/s41572-020-0147-3

[7] Nyaruaba R, Okoye CO, Akan OD, Mwaliko C, Ebido CC, Ayoola A, et al. Socio-economic impacts of emerging infectious diseases in Africa. Infectious diseases (London, England). 2022;**54**(5):315-324. DOI: 10.1080/23744235.2021.2022195

[8] Di Bari C, Venkateswaran N, Fastl C, Gabriël S, Grace D, Havelaar AH, et al. The global burden of neglected zoonotic diseases: Current state of evidence. One Health. 2023;**17**:100595. DOI: 10.1016/j.onehlt.2023.100595

[9] WHO. WHO Technical Guidance Notes on Sendai Framework Reporting for Ministries of Health. Geneva, Switzerland: World Health Organization; 2020

[10] Welburn S, Beange I, Ducrotoy M, Okello A. The neglected zoonoses--the case for integrated control and advocacy. Clinical Microbiology and Infection : The Official Publication of the European Society of Clinical Microbiology and Infectious Diseases. 2015;**21**(5):433-443. DOI: 10.1016/j.cmi.2015.04.011

[11] Weld ED, Waitt C, Barnes K, Garcia Bournissen F. Twice neglected? Neglected diseases in neglected populations. British Journal of Clinical Pharmacology. 2022;**88**(2):367-373. DOI: 10.1111/bcp.15148

[12] Ayouba A, Mbala-Kingebeni P, Keita A, Vidal N, Lacroix A, Touré A, et al. New technologies for controlling emerging infectious diseases in Guinea and the Democratic Republic of the Congo: Their role in response to the Ebola epidemic. Médecine et Santé Tropicales. 2019;**29**(4):362-365. DOI: 10.1684/mst.2019.0942

[13] Beda E, Karimuribo ED, Sayalel K, Short N, Wambura P, Mboera LG, et al. Towards one health disease surveillance: The southern African Centre for infectious disease surveillance approach.

The Onderstepoort Journal of Veterinary Research. 2012;**79**(2):454. DOI: 10.4102/ojvr.v79i2.454

[14] Chauhan RP, Dessie ZG, Noreddin A, El Zowalaty ME. Systematic review of important viral diseases in Africa in light of the 'one health' concept. Pathogens. 2020;**9**(4):1-83. DOI: 10.3390/pathogens9040301

[15] Massengo NRB, Tinto B, Simonin Y. One health approach to arbovirus control in Africa: Interests, challenges, and difficulties. Microorganisms. 2023;**11**(6):1496. DOI: 10.3390/microorganisms11061496

[16] Monday B, Gitta SN, Wasswa P, et al. Paradigm shift: Contribution of field epidemiology training in advancing the "one health" approach to strengthen disease surveillance and outbreak investigations in Africa. The Pan African Medical Journal. 2011;**10**(Suppl 1):13

[17] Mumba SO. Analysis of Factors Influencing Multi-Sectoral Collaboration in Responding to Emerging Zoonotic Diseases: A Case of Kilosa District Council. Dar es Salaam, Tanzania: Tanzania Muhimbili University of Health and Allied Sciences; 2017

[18] Rweyemamu MM, Paweska J, Kambarage D, Namuba F. Towards one Africa, one health: The southern African Centre for Infectious Disease Surveillance one Health focus on infectious diseases. Onderstepoort Journal of Veterinary Research. 2012;**79**(2):1-2. DOI: 10.4102/ojvr.v79i2.449

[19] Tajudeen YA, Oladipo HJ, Oladunjoye IO, Yusuf RO, Sodiq H, Omotosho AO, et al. Emerging arboviruses of public health concern in Africa: Priorities for future research and control strategies. Challenges. 2022;**13**(2):60. DOI: 10.3390/challe13020060

[20] Mbim EN, Edet UO, Okoroiwu HU, Nwaokorie FO, Edet AE, Owolabi A, et al. Arbovirus and its potential to lead the next global pandemic from sub-Saharan Africa: What lessons have we learned from COVID-19? Germs. 2022;**12**(4):538. DOI: 10.18683/germs.2022.1358

[21] Chor K, Medycznego U, Indyjskiego O, Zjednoczonych S. Gorączka chikungunya. Reumatologia. 2011;**49**(6):439-445

[22] Chattopadhyay A, Aguilar PV, Bopp NE, Yarovinsky TO, Weaver SC, Rose JK. A recombinant virus vaccine that protects against both chikungunya and Zika virus infections. Vaccine. 2018;**36**(27):3894-3900. DOI: 10.1016/j.vaccine.2018.05.095

[23] Lu H, Stratton CW, Tang YW. Outbreak of pneumonia of unknown etiology in Wuhan, China: The mystery and the miracle. Journal of Medical Virology. 2020;**92**(4):401-402. DOI: 10.1002/jmv.25678

[24] Abdullahi AM. Virology and epidemiology of the 2019 coronavirus disease (Covid-19). Journal of Community Medicine and Public Health Reports Virology. 2020;**1**(1):1-8. DOI: 10.38207/jcmphr20213

[25] Waterman SH, Gubler DJ. Dengue fever. Clinics in Dermatology. 1989;**7**(1):117-122. DOI: 10.1016/0738-081x(89)90034-5

[26] Johnson KM. Ebola haemorrhagic fever in Zaire, 1976. Bulletin of the World Health Organization. 1978;**56**(2):271-293

[27] WHO. Ebola virus disease in West Africa, the first 9 months of the

epidemic and forward projections. The New England Journal of Medicine. 2014;**371**(16):1481-1495. DOI: 10.1056/NEJMoa1411100

[28] Von Magnus P, Andersen EA, Petersen KB, Birch-Andersen A. A pox-like disease in cynomolgus monkeys. Acta Path Microbiol Scand. 1959;**46**:156-176

[29] Zumla A, Valdoleiros SR, Haider N, Asogun D, Ntoumi F, Petersen E, et al. Monkeypox outbreaks outside endemic regions: Scientific and social priorities. The Lancet. Infectious Diseases. 2022;**22**(7):929-931. DOI: 10.1016/S1473-3099(22)00354-1

[30] Bonavita CM, Wells HL, Anthony SJ. Cellular dynamics shape recombination frequency in coronaviruses. PLoS Pathogens. 2024;**20**(9):e1012596. DOI: 10.1371/journal.ppat.1012596

[31] Towner JS, Khristova ML, Sealy TK, Vincent MJ, Erickson BR, Bawiec DA, et al. Marburgvirus genomics and association with a large hemorrhagic fever outbreak in Angola. Journal of Virology. 2006;**80**. DOI: 10.1128/jvi.00069-06

[32] Monath TP. A short history of Lassa fever: The first 10-15 years after discovery. Current Opinion in Virology. 2019;**37**:77-83. DOI: 10.1016/j.coviro.2019.06.005

[33] Zhao S, Musa SS, Fu H, He D, Qin J. Large-scale Lassa fever outbreaks in Nigeria: Quantifying the association between disease reproduction number and local rainfall. Epidemiology and Infection. 2020;**148**:e4. DOI: 10.1017/S0950268819002267

[34] Dick GW, Kitchen SF, Haddow AJ. Zika virus. I. Isolations and serological specificity. Transactions of the Royal Society of Tropical Medicine and Hygiene. 1952;**46**(5):509-520. DOI: 10.1016/0035-9203(52)90042-4

[35] WHO. Report of a WHO Meeting on Skin-Related Neglected Tropical Diseases in West Africa, Geneva, 3-5 October 2022. Geneva, Switzerland: World Health Organization; 2023b

[36] Adam A, Jassoy C. Epidemiology and laboratory diagnostics of dengue, yellow fever, Zika, and chikungunya virus infections in Africa. Pathogens. 2021;**10**(10):1324. DOI: 10.3390/pathogens10101324

[37] LaBrunda M, Amin N. The emerging threat of Ebola. In: Global Health Security: Recognizing Vulnerabilities, Creating Opportunities. Cham, Switzerland: Springer Publishing International; 2020. pp. 103-139. DOI: 10.1007/978-3-030-23491-1_6

[38] WHO. Ebola Virus Disease Democratic Republic of Congo: External Situation Report. 2019. p. 34

[39] Leroy EM, Kumulungui B, Pourrut X, Rouquet P, Hassanin A, Yaba P, et al. Fruit bats as reservoirs of Ebola virus. Nature. 2005;**438**(7068):575-576. DOI: 10.1038/438575a

[40] Leroy EM, Epelboin A, Mondonge V, Pourrut X, Gonzalez J-P, Muyembe-Tamfum J-J, et al. Human Ebola outbreak resulting from direct exposure to fruit bats in Luebo, Democratic Republic of Congo, 2007. Vector-Borne and Zoonotic Diseases. 2009;**9**(6):723-728. DOI: 10.1089/vbz.2008.0167

[41] Ogbu O, Ajuluchukwu E, Uneke CJ. Lassa fever in West African sub-region : An overview. Journal of Vector Borne Diseases. 2007;**44**(March):1-11

[42] Happi AN, Olumade TJ, Ogunsanya OA, Sijuwola AE,

Ogunleye SC, Oguzie JU, et al. Increased prevalence of Lassa fever virus-positive rodents and diversity of infected species found during human Lassa fever epidemics in Nigeria. Microbiology Spectrum. 2022;**10**(4):e0036622. DOI: 10.1128/spectrum.00366-22

[43] Abdulhamid A, Hussaini N, Musa SS, He D. Results in physics: Mathematical analysis of the Lassa fever epidemic with effects of environmental transmission. Results in Physics. 2022;**35**(February):105335. DOI: 10.1016/j.rinp.2022.105335

[44] Akhmetzhanov AR, Asai Y, Nishiura H. Quantifying the seasonal drivers of transmission for Lassa fever in Nigeria. Philosophical Transactions of the Royal Society B. 2019;**374**(1775):20180268. DOI: 10.1098/rstb.2018.0268

[45] Barua S, Dénes A, Ibrahim MA. A seasonal model to assess intervention strategies for preventing periodic recurrence of Lassa fever. Heliyon. 2021;**7**(8):13-22. DOI: 10.1016/j.heliyon.2021.e07760

[46] Uchenna Emeribe A, Nasir Abdullahi I, OR Ajagbe O, Egede Ugwu C, Oloche Onoja S, Dahiru Abubakar S, et al. Incidence, drivers and global health implications of the 2019/2020 yellow fever sporadic outbreaks in sub-Saharan Africa. Pathogens and Disease. 2021;**79**(4):ftab017

[47] Robertson SE, Hull BP, Tomori O, Bele O, LeDuc JW, Esteves K. Yellow fever: A decade of reemergence. Yellow fever: A decade of reemergence. JAMA. 1996;**276**(14):1157-1162

[48] Findlay GM, Kirk R, MacCallum FO. Yellow fever and the Anglo-Egyptian Sudan: Distribution of immune bodies to yellow fever. Annals of Tropical Medicine & Parasitology. 1941;**35**(2):121-139. DOI: 10.1080/00034983.1941.11685117

[49] Mutebi J, Barrett ADT. The epidemiology of yellow fever in Africa. Microbes and Infections. 2002;**4**(*14*):1459-1468. DOI: 10.1016/S1286-4579(02)00028-X

[50] CDC. Ebola outbreak updates; 2020. Available from: www.cdc.gov

[51] Bunge ME, Hoet B, Chen L, Lienert F, Weidenthaler H, Baer RL, et al. The changing epidemiology of human monkeypox — A potential threat ? A systematic review. PLoS Neglected Tropical Diseases. 2022;**16**(2):1-20. DOI: 10.1371/journal.pntd.0010141

[52] Ladnyj I, Ziegler P, Kima E. A human infection caused by monkeypox virus in Basankusu territory, Democratic Republic of the Congo. Bulletin of the World Health Organization. 1972;**46**(5):593-597

[53] WHO. MonkeyPox in Africa Region. 2024. Available from: https://www.who.int/emergencies/disease-outbreak-news/item/2024-DON528

[54] Ndembi N, Folayan MO, Komakech A, Mercy K, Tessema S, Mbala-Kingebeni P, et al. Evolving epidemiology of Mpox in Africa in 2024. The New England Journal of Medicine. 2025;**392**(7):666-676. DOI: 10.1056/NEJMoa2411368

[55] Sklenovská N, Van Ranst M. Emergence of Monkeypox as the Most important Orthopoxvirus infection in humans. Frontiers in Public Health. 2018;**6**:241. DOI: 10.3389/fpubh.2018.00241

[56] Bird BH, Ksiazek TG, Nichol ST, Maclachlan NJ. Rift valley fever virus.

Journal of the American Veterinary Medical Association. 2009;**234**(7):883-893. DOI: 10.2460/javma.234.7.883

[57] Messina JP, Brady OJ, Golding N, Kraemer MUG, Wint GRW, Ray SE, et al. The current and future global distribution and population. Nature Microbiology. 2019;**4**(September 2019):1508-1515. DOI: 10.1038/s41564-019-0476-8

[58] Roy SK, Bhattacharjee S. Dengue virus: Epidemiology, biology, and disease aetiology. Canadian Journal of Microbiology. 2021;**67**(10):687-702. DOI: 10.1139/cjm-2020-0572

[59] WHO. Multi-country Outbreak of Dengue Benin, Burkina Faso, Cabo Verde, Chad, Côte d'Ivoire, Ethiopia, Ghana, Guinea, Mali, Mauritius, Niger, Nigeria, São Tomé and Príncipe, Senegal, and Togo Consolidated Regional Situation Repo. 2024. Available from: https://iris.who.int/bitstream/handle/10665/376307/AFRO.Dengue.Sitrep004-20240303.pdf?sequence=1

[60] Teurlai M, Menkès CE, Cavarero V, Degallier N, Descloux E, Grangeon J-P, et al. Socio-economic and climate factors associated with dengue fever spatial heterogeneity: A worked example in New Caledonia. PLoS Neglected Tropical Diseases. 2015;**9**(12):e0004211. DOI: 10.1371/journal.pntd.0004211

[61] UNAIDS. Global and Regional Data. 2021

[62] Ekholuenetale M, Owobi OU, Barrow A. Achieving the UNAIDS first '95'in prenuptial HIV/AIDS testing among reproductive-aged Rwandese women: A multilevel analysis of 2019-20 population-based data. PLOS Global Public Health. 2023;**3**(2):e0001033. DOI: 10.1371/journal.pgph.0001033

[63] WHO. HIV/AIDS in Africa Region. 2023. Available from: https://www.afro.who.int/health-topics/hivaids

[64] Blach S, Zeuzem S, Manns M, Altraif I, Duberg A-S, Muljono HD, et al. Global prevalence and genotype distribution of hepatitis C virus infection in 2015 : A modelling study. The Lancet Gastroenterology & Hepatology. 2017;**2**:161-176. DOI: 10.1016/S2468-1253(16)30181-9

[65] Lavanchy D. Evolving epidemiology of hepatitis C virus. Clinical Microbiology and Infection. 2011;**17**(2):107-115. DOI: 10.1111/j.1469-0691.2010.03432.x

[66] WHO. Hepatitis C. 2024. Available from: https://www.who.int/publications/i/item/9789240091672

[67] Seu R, Riback LR, Nyakowa M, Lizcano J, Musyoki H, Ross J, et al. Challenges and best practices for hepatitis C care among people who inject drugs in resource limited settings: Focus group discussions with healthcare providers in Kenya. Global Public Health. 2022;**17**(12):3627-3637. DOI: 10.1080/17441692.2022.2110919

[68] Salomon I, Olivier S, Egide N. Advancing hepatitis C elimination in Africa: Insights from Egypt. Hepatic Medicine : Evidence And Research. 2024;**16**:37-44. DOI: 10.2147/hmer.S470344

[69] Carruthers VB, Cotter PA, Kumamoto CA. Microbial pathogenesis: Mechanisms of infectious disease. Cell Host & Microbe. 2007;**2**(4):214-219. DOI: 10.1016/j.chom.2007.09.007

[70] Savić S, Vidić B, Grgić Z, Potkonjak A, Spasojevic L. Emerging vector-borne diseases–incidence through vectors. Frontiers in Public

Health. 2014;**2**:267. DOI: 10.3389/fpubh.2014.00267

[71] Lindsay SW, Wilson A, Golding N, Scott TW, Takken W. Improving the built environment in urban areas to control Aedes aegypti-borne diseases. Bulletin of the World Health Organization. 2017;**95**(8):607. DOI: 10.2471/BLT.16.189688

[72] Pearce JC, Learoyd TP, Langendorf BJ, Logan JG. Japanese encephalitis: The vectors, ecology and potential for expansion. Journal of Travel Medicine. 2018;**25**(suppl_1):S16-S26. DOI: 10.1093/jtm/tay009

[73] Kayondo SP, Byamugisha JK, Ntuyo P. Prevalence of hepatitis B virus infection and associated risk factors among pregnant women attending antenatal clinic in Mulago hospital, Uganda: A cross-sectional study. BMJ Open. 2020;**10**(6):e033043. DOI: 10.1136/bmjopen-2019-033043

[74] Guure C, Obiri-Yeboah Laryea SM, Dery S, Baptista da Silva C, Asamoah-Adu C, Ayisi-Addo S, et al. Behavioural risk for HIV, hepatitis B, and hepatitis C infections among a population of drug users and injectors across four regions in Ghana. Interdiscip Perspect Infectious Disease. 2022;**2022**:2544481. DOI: 10.1155/2022/2544481

[75] Manguvo A, Mafuvadze B. The impact of traditional and religious practices on the spread of Ebola in West Africa: Time for a strategic shift. The Pan African Medical Journal. 2015;**22**(Suppl 1):9. DOI: 10.11694/pamj.supp.2015.22.1.6190

[76] Ka-Wai Hui E. Reasons for the increase in emerging and re-emerging viral infectious diseases. Microbes and Infection. 2019;**8**(3):905-916. DOI: 10.1016/j.micinf.2005.06.032

[77] Sattar SA, Jason T, Bidawid S, Farber J. Foodborne spread of hepatitis a: Recent studies on virus survival, transfer and inactivation. Canadian Journal of Infectious Diseases. 2000;**11**(3):159-163. DOI: 10.1155/2000/805156

[78] Rulli MC, Santini M, Hayman DT, D'Odorico P. The nexus between forest fragmentation in Africa and Ebola virus disease outbreaks. Scientific Reports. 2017;**7**(1):41613. DOI: 10.1038/srep41613

[79] Alexander KA, Sanderson CE, Marathe M, Lewis BL, Rivers CM, Shaman J, et al. What factors might have led to the emergence of Ebola in West Africa? PLoS Neglected Tropical Diseases. 2015;**9**(6):e0003652. DOI: 10.1371/journal.pntd.0003652

[80] Epstein JH, Field HE, Luby S, Pulliam JR, Daszak P. Nipah virus: Impact, origins, and causes of emergence. Current Infectious Disease Reports. 2006;**8**(1):59-65. DOI: 10.1007/s11908-006-0036-2

[81] Looi LM, Chua KB. Lessons from the Nipah virus outbreak in Malaysia. Malaysian Journal of Pathology. 2007;**29**(2):63-67

[82] Johnson KM. Emerging viruses in context: An overview of viral haemorrhagic fevers. Emerging Viruses. 2011:45-57

[83] Hassan OA, Ahlm C, Sang R, Evander M. The 2007 Rift Valley fever outbreak in Sudan. PLoS Neglected Tropical Diseases. 2011;**5**(9):e1229. DOI: 10.1371/journal.pntd.0001229

[84] Khabbaz R, Bell BP, Schuchat A, Ostroff SM, Moseley R, Levitt A, et al. Emerging and reemerging infectious disease threats. Mandell, Douglas, and Bennett's principles and practice of infectious diseases.

2014;**158-177**:e6. DOI: 10.1016/B978-1-4557-4801-3.00014-X

[85] Rohr JR, Barrett CB, Civitello DJ, Craft ME, Delius B, DeLeo GA, et al. Emerging human infectious diseases and the links to global food production. Nature Sustainability. 2019;**2**(6):445-456. DOI: 10.1038/s41893-019-0293-3

[86] Chakrabartty I, Khan M, Mahanta S, Chopra H, Dhawan M, Choudhary OP, et al. Comparative overview of emerging RNA viruses: Epidemiology, pathogenesis, diagnosis, and current treatment. Annals of Medicine and Surgery (Lond). 2022;**79**:103985. DOI: 10.1016/j.amsu.2022.103985

[87] Domingo E. Quasispecies and RNA Virus Evolution: Principles and Consequences. Vol. 14. Austin, Texas: Landes Bioscience; 2001

[88] Ka-Wai Hui E. Reasons for the increase in emerging and re-emerging viral infectious diseases. Microbes and Infection. 2006;**8**(3):905-916. DOI: 10.1016/j.micinf.2005.06.032

[89] Hatta M, Gao P, Halfmann P, Kawaoka Y. Molecular basis for high virulence of Hong Kong H5N1 influenza a viruses. Science. 2001;**293**(5536):1840-1842. DOI: 10.1126/science.1062882

[90] Worobey M, Holmes EC. Evolutionary aspects of recombination in RNA viruses. Journal of General Virology. 2000;**80**(10):2535-2543. DOI: 10.1099/0022-1317-80-10-2535

[91] Ahmed SM, Hall AJ, Robinson AE, Verhoef L, Premkumar P, Parashar UD, et al. Global prevalence of norovirus in cases of gastroenteritis: A systematic review and meta-analysis. The Lancet Infectious Diseases. 2014;**14**(8):725-730. DOI: 10.1016/S1473-3099(14)70767-4

[92] Shenge JA, Opayele AV. The impact and control of emerging and Re-emerging viral diseases in the environment: An African perspective. In: Current Microbiological Research in Africa: Selected Applications for Sustainable Environmental Management. Cham, Switzerland: Springer Publishing International; 2020. pp. 185-202. DOI: 10.1007/978-3-030-35296-7_7

[93] Cassadou S, Boucau S, Petit-Sinturel M, Huc P, Leparc-Goffart I, Ledrans M. Emergence of chikungunya fever on the French side of Saint Martin island, October to December 2013. Eurosurveillance. 2014;**19**(13):20752. DOI: 10.2807/1560-7917.es2014.19.13.20752

[94] Nash D, Mostashari F, Fine A, Miller J, O'leary D, Murray K, et al. The outbreak of West Nile virus infection in the New York City area in 1999. New England Journal of Medicine. 2001;**344**(24):1807-1814. DOI: 10.1056/NEJM200106143442401

[95] Mandyata CB, Olowski LK, Mutale W. Challenges of implementing the integrated disease surveillance and response strategy in Zambia: A health worker perspective. BMC Public Health. 2017;**17**:1-12. DOI: 10.1186/s12889-017-4791-9

[96] Phalkey RK, Yamamoto S, Awate P, Marx M. Challenges with the implementation of an integrated disease surveillance and response (IDSR) system: Systematic review of the lessons learned. Health Policy and Planning. 2013;**30**(1):131-143. DOI: 10.1093/heapol/czt097

[97] Nakiire L, Masiira B, Kihembo C, Katushabe E, Natseri N, Nabukenya I, et al. Healthcare workers' experiences regarding scaling up of training on integrated disease surveillance and

response (IDSR) in Uganda, 2016: Cross sectional qualitative study. BMC Health Services Research. 2019;**19**:1-9. DOI: 10.1186/s12913-019-3923-6

[98] Zinsstag J, Schelling E, Wyss K, Mahamat MB. Potential of cooperation between human and animal health to strengthen health systems. The Lancet. 2005;**366**(9503):2142-2145. DOI: 10.1016/S0140-6736(05)67731-8

[99] Zinsstag J, Schelling E, Waltner-Toews D, Tanner M. From "one medicine" to "one health" and systemic approaches to health and well-being. Preventive Veterinary Medicine. 2011;**101**(3-4):148-156. DOI: 10.1016/j.prevetmed.2010.07.003

[100] Morens DM, Fauci AS. Emerging infectious diseases in 2012: 20 years after the institute of medicine report. MBio. 2012;**3**(6):1-4. DOI: 10.1128/mBio.00494-12

[101] Cascio A, Bosilkovski M, Rodriguez-Morales AJ, Pappas G. The socio-ecology of zoonotic infections. Clinical Microbiology and Infection. 2011;**17**(3):336-342. DOI: 10.1111/j.1469-0691.2010.03451.x

[102] Engering A, Hogerwerf L, Slingenbergh J. Pathogen–host–environment interplay and disease emergence. Emerging Microbes & Infections. 2013;**2**(2):e5. DOI: 10.1038/emi.2013.5

[103] Kilpatrick AM, Randolph SE. Drivers, dynamics, and control of emerging vector-borne zoonotic diseases. The Lancet. 2012;**380**(9857):1946-1955. DOI: 10.1016/S0140-6736(12)61151-9

[104] Karesh WB, Dobson A, Lloyd-Smith JO, Lubroth J, Dixon MA, Bennett M, et al. Ecology of zoonoses: Natural and unnatural histories. Lancet. 2012;**380**(9857):1936-1945. DOI: 10.1016/s0140-6736(12)61678-x

[105] WHO. One Health in Action: What Wildlife Health Surveillance Can Tell Us About Pandemic Prevention. 2024. Available from: https://www.who.int/westernpacific/newsroom/feature-stories/item/one-health-in-action--what-wildlife-health-surveillance-can-tell-us-about-pandemic-prevention

[106] Daszak P, Cunningham AA, Hyatt AD. Emerging infectious diseases of wildlife--threats to biodiversity and human health. Science. 2000;**287**(5452):443-449. DOI: 10.1126/science.287.5452.443

[107] Morse SS, Mazet JA, Woolhouse M, Parrish CR, Carroll D, Karesh WB, et al. Prediction and prevention of the next pandemic zoonosis. The Lancet. 2012;**380**(9857):1956-1965. DOI: 10.1016/S0140-6736(12)61684-5

[108] Grace D, Mutua F, Ochungo P, Kruska R, Jones K, Brierley L, et al. Mapping of poverty and likely zoonoses hotspots. In: Zoonoses Project 4. Report to the UK Department for International Development. Nairobi, Kenya: ILRI; 2012

[109] Hasanov E, Zeynalova S, Geleishvili M, Maes E, Tongren E, Marshall E, et al. Assessing the impact of public education on a preventable zoonotic disease: Rabies. Epidemiology and Infection. 2018;**146**(2):227-235. DOI: 10.1017/s0950268817002850

[110] Chomel BB, Boulouis H-J, Breitschwerdt EB, Kasten RW, Vayssier-Taussat M, Birtles RJ, et al. Ecological fitness and strategies of adaptation of Bartonella species to their hosts and vectors. Veterinary Research. 2009;**40**(2):29. DOI: 10.1051/vetres/2009011

[111] Lunney JK, Benfield DA, Rowland RR. Porcine reproductive and respiratory syndrome virus: An update on an emerging and re-emerging viral disease of swine. Virus Research. 2010;**154**(1-2):1-6. DOI: 10.1016/j.virusres.2010.10.009

[112] Jones KE, Patel NG, Levy MA, Storeygard A, Balk D, Gittleman JL, et al. Global trends in emerging infectious diseases. Nature. 2008;**451**(7181):990-993. DOI: 10.1038/nature06536

[113] WHO. Taking a multisectoral one health approach: A tripartite guide to addressing zoonotic diseases in countries. Food & Agriculture Org; 2019